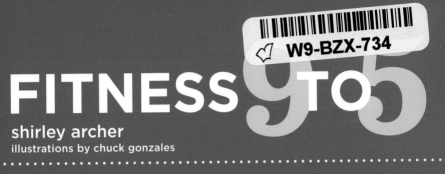

FITNESS 9 TO 5

shirley archer
illustrations by chuck gonzales

easy exercises for the working week

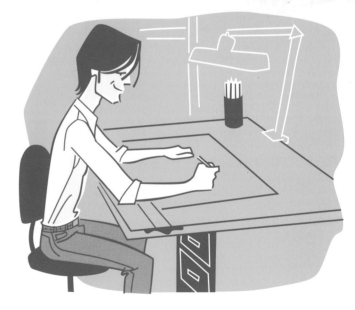

CHRONICLE BOOKS
SAN FRANCISCO

This book is dedicated to all those who work hard in the office to earn a living and who want to be healthy and fit. You deserve to have it all.

Text copyright © 2006 by Shirley Archer.
Illustrations copyright © 2006 by Chuck Gonzales.

Library of Congress Cataloging-in-Publication Data available.

ISBN 0-8118-4874-4

Manufactured in China.

Designed by Ph.D.

Distributed in Canada by Raincoast Books
9050 Shaughnessy Street
Vancouver, British Columbia V6P 6E5

10 9 8 7 6 5 4 3 2 1

Chronicle Books LLC
85 Second Street
San Francisco, California 94105

www.chroniclebooks.com

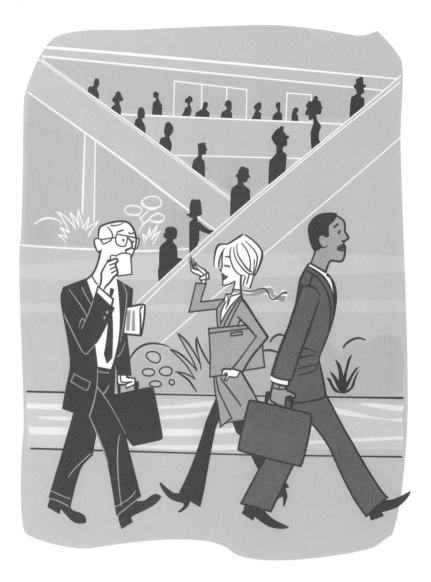

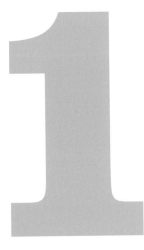

Office Fitness
For Every Body:
An Introduction

Of course you don't have time to go to the gym for an hour every day. Like most of us, you have to earn a living. Yet, as you sit at your desk, you feel your tushie spreading, your neck and shoulders aching. You know that you need to do something. But what can you do?

You can work out at the office, that's what you can do! *Fitness 9 to 5* shows you how to tone up, trim down, and improve your health by incorporating exercises into your daily work routine. Do these exercises at your desk, at the board meeting, or while taking calls. You don't even have to suit up. You can do all of these exercises while dressed in your business clothes.

If you're thinking that this sort of exercise program sounds too good or too silly to be true, that it could never work, consider this: How many times have you paid for a gym membership only to discover that you're never able to go? How many times have you set your alarm for an early workout, only to fall asleep in the middle of the morning at your desk? How many times have you tried to work out at the end of the day, only to find yourself too tired and too hungry to do anything other than shuffle home, eat, and sit on the couch? It happens to all of us. The beauty of *Fitness 9 to 5* is that you don't have to go to the gym. You don't have to add another item to your already full calendar. Instead, you're integrating exercise into your everyday routine. You're maximizing your time. You're multitasking.

Sure, it's great to go to the gym or work with a personal trainer. And if you can do that a few days of the week, that's fantastic. But on those days when deadlines are calling and you can't leave the office, you'll benefit greatly from the exercises outlined in *Fitness 9 to 5*. Never underestimate the power of increasing your daily activities to help you feel better and lose weight. Some exercise is always better than none. Technology today makes it much too easy for us to sit for hours. Our minds are busy, but our bodies are still. We need to stand up, walk away from our seats, and take back the power of our legs.

The World Health Organization recommends that people throughout the world move more to improve health. The American College of Sports Medicine and the U.S. Surgeon General suggest that you do a minimum amount of physical activity to improve and maintain your endurance and to reduce disease risks, especially that of heart disease. Studies show that you can reap health benefits simply from being moderately active for at least thirty minutes, or for three ten-minute bouts, on five or more days of the week. It's that easy!

Of course, more exercise will improve your fitness level; this guideline refers to the minimum amount of time you need to invest for better health. Moderate activity includes climbing stairs, walking to the office, performing light calisthenics, and weight training. Doing the exercises daily in *Fitness 9 to 5*—such as the Performance-Maximizing Parking Lot Stroll and the No-Limits Stairwell Bun Blaster—meets these government guidelines for physical activity and improves your health. You will get results!

The exercises in *Fitness 9 to 5* also help you tone up and stretch out so that you look and feel great. Strength-training exercises include moves such as Early-Bird Coffeepot Curls to tone your arms and "I'm Not Quite Ready to Work!" Chair Squats to firm up your behind. Stretches like the commuting Crawling-Bus Neck Rolls and the Sit-Up-and-Succeed Chest and Shoulder Opener release tension and help prevent back pain.

Each exercise is described in simple steps and includes revealing information on how many calories are burned over the course of a year simply by doing the exercises daily at the office. These calorie counts are not to turn you into an obsessive-compulsive calorie counter; rather, the counts illustrate the power of adding a few moves daily that help you manage your weight, tone up, and feel great. For example, if you undertook just five of the more challenging exercises five days a week for a year, your total additional calories burned could be 17,500! If you did not change any of your eating habits, that additional calorie burn could result in as many as five pounds lost over a year. If you did sixty-five exercises five days a week for a year, you could work off as much as twenty-nine pounds.

Keep in mind that you burn approximately one calorie per minute just by sitting and breathing. The goal, then, is to find a way to squeeze in small activities during your day to use more energy. The calories burned are based on an average 150- to 160-pound person, so individual results will vary. We understand you need to accomplish work at the office as well, so consider how incorporating even a few exercises can make a powerful impact.

Everybody knows that feeling great is not just about exercise—it's about creating a healthier lifestyle. To inspire you to keep up the good work, this book includes lots of motivating and practical tips. These ideas help you to increase your minute-by-minute caloric burn, to improve your workday wellness, and to beat on-the-job stress. Remember, a healthier and stronger you leads to more productivity, better relationships, and higher-quality work in the long term. Your well-being is worth the extra commitment required to make adding some healthy habits a priority.

For ease of reference, the book is organized chronologically, with suggestions for exercises to do throughout the day—from before you get out of bed in the morning to your commute back home. All exercises are clearly explained and illustrated—you're even given practical ideas of when to fit them into your daily routine. The only missing ingredient is you.

Before you start with this, or any exercise program, make sure that you are healthy enough to exercise. If you're a beginner, start slow, take it easy, and progress gradually. Most of us get excited when we begin something new. People commonly do too much, too soon. To avoid this, these exercises are broken down into small, achievable portions. Do what you can and you will see improvements. Give yourself time. Start with ten minutes a day and work up to thirty minutes or more. Never do anything that causes you pain. Before you know it, the flight of stairs that used to feel challenging and leave you breathless to climb will feel easy and comfortable.

This workout is convenient and does not require fancy equipment. For walking and stair-climbing, keep a pair of comfortable, flat walking shoes in the office. Your shoes will always be handy, and you won't have to worry about bringing them to work. For a few of the back- and shoulder-toning moves, you can use an inexpensive, four-foot, elastic resistance band. For a few of the lower-body exercises, you can use an ankle weight. For other toning exercises, like reverse biceps curls, you can use a water bottle filled to the amount of weight that you can lift. As you become stronger, increase the amount of water in the bottle to increase the challenge.

The stretches, too, require no extra equipment. However, if you're prone to stiffness, a strap is a helpful tool. I recommend a multiple-loop strap to make it easier to adjust the stretch. As you exercise, breathe deeply and avoid holding your breath. Relax and release any excess tension in your body, especially in the neck, shoulders, and jaw. Remember good posture when you're standing, sitting, walking, climbing stairs, or performing any of the toning moves. If you are wearing high heels, simply slip off your shoes before doing standing exercises like squats. I repeat, avoid anything that causes pain.

Recruit a buddy in your office to help you stick with the exercises to get even better results. Studies show that one of the best ways to keep up with a new exercise program is to have the support of people around you. See if a friend in your office will work with you. Arrange to do fitness lunch walks together, meet in the stairwell, and keep each other motivated.

This exercise guide provides a unique and innovative way to get in shape, stay healthy, *and* keep your job. Who says you can't have it all? You can. Don't wait. Start today.

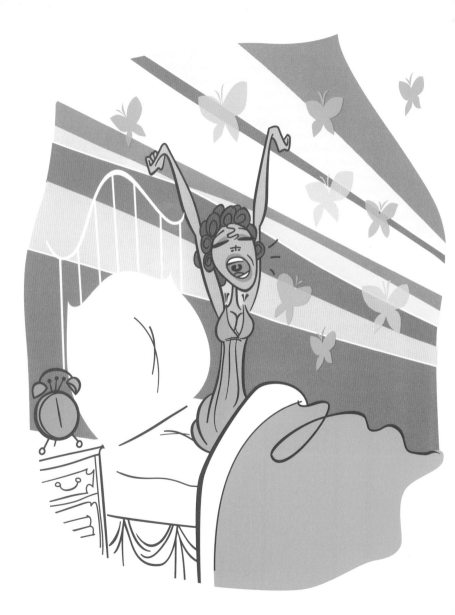

prework workouts

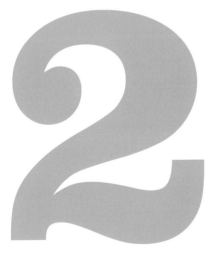

1. embrace-the-day knee-hug stretch

Start your day feeling fresh. Enjoy gentle stretches that relieve early morning stiffness so you can begin moving easily and breathing deeply.

> Lie on your back in bed.

> Place your hands around the backs of your thighs as you move your knees toward your chest.

> Inhale for four to five seconds as you hold the position.

> Exhale for five to six seconds as you gently draw your knees closer to your chest. Feel the stretch in your buttocks and lower back.

> Hold for at least three breath cycles, breathing in deeply and exhaling completely. One inhalation and one exhalation equal one breath cycle.

VARIATION

For a more gentle stretch, draw one knee toward your chest at a time. Follow directions at left. Repeat with other leg.

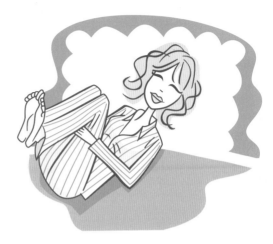

SECRETS OF SUCCESS

Move through a comfortable range of motion only. Avoid any feelings of pain or strain. Breathe deeply in and out through your nose. Release tension throughout your body as you exhale.

One minute of stretching burns 3.2 calories.

ONE YEAR

3.2 calories x 5 days per week = 16 calories

16 calories x 50 weeks per year = 800 calories

800 calories ÷ 3,500 calories per pound = .23 pound

By adding one minute of early morning stretches per day, you can burn off almost ¼ pound per year.

2. seize-the-moment reverse curls and crunches

It's never too early for an ab workout. Who needs coffee? Get your blood pumping with this quickie A.M. set instead. Get in the habit of sneaking in bits of exercise whenever an opportunity presents itself. All those minutes add up!

> Lie on your back in bed. If you have a particularly soft mattress, you may want to do this exercise on the floor.

> Place your fingertips behind your head with your elbows out wide so your arms are in a diamond shape.

> Bend your knees approximately 90 degrees, feet elevated, shoulders relaxed.

> Exhale as you contract your abdominal muscles and draw your knees up toward your chest, lifting your lower spine off the mattress. Draw your abdominals in toward your spine. Keep your upper body relaxed.

> Inhale as you lower your hips to the starting position.

> Do twelve repetitions.

> Switch the focus to lifting your chest, keeping your knees bent and feet elevated.

> **Exhale as you curl your upper body,
> bringing your lower ribs toward
> your pelvis. Feel your abdominal
> muscles contract.**

> **Do twelve repetitions.**

One minute of toning exercises burns 5.5 calories.

ONE YEAR

5.5 calories x 5 days per week = 27.5 calories

27.5 calories x 50 weeks per year = 1,375 calories

1,375 calories ÷ 3,500 calories per pound = .39 pound

By adding one minute of toning exercises per day, you can burn off approximately
3/8 pound per year.

3. take-on-the-day side torso stretch

Wake up your entire body with this full-length stretch. Then, roll out of bed and start your day feeling good about yourself.

> Lie on your back in bed.

> Reach your arms over your head. Hold your hands loosely together. Inhale.

> Exhale as you slide your body to the side into a crescent shape. Inhale as you hold the position.

> Exhale for five to six seconds, lengthening your hipbone away from your lowest rib. Feel the stretch along the side of your torso.

> Hold for at least three breath cycles, breathing deeply and exhaling completely.

> Relax and return to center.

> Repeat on the other side.

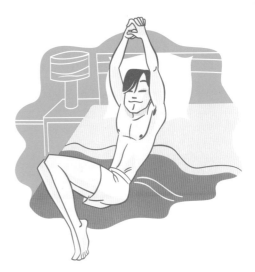

One minute of stretching burns 3.2 calories.

ONE YEAR

3.2 calories x 5 days per week = 16 calories

16 calories x 50 weeks per year = 800 calories

800 calories ÷ 3,500 calories per pound = .23 pound

By adding one minute of early morning stretches per day, you can burn off almost $1/4$ pound per year.

4. every-minute-counts car-seat posture check and ab toner

Don't waste time getting angry and agitated. Use that energy to feel great about yourself instead. Be positive and use the precious time when you're caught in gridlock to improve your posture and tone your abs.

> Sit in your car seat on your sitz bones with your legs at right angles and space behind your knees. Avoid pressing the backs of your legs against any of your seats or chairs as it can impair circulation.

> Place your feet hip-width apart. Put your foot on the brake pedal; keep your hips parallel to the dashboard.

> Draw your abdominal muscles inward. Adjust the car seat to support the natural curve in your lower back.

> Lift your breastbone upward and draw your lower rib cage inward; align your shoulders above your hips.

> Relax your shoulders. Adjust the steering wheel so your arms hang naturally at your sides when your hands are on the wheel.

> Align your ears above your shoulders and keep your chin level. Adjust your headrest.

> Inhale deeply, keeping your shoulders low and relaxed.

- Exhale completely, drawing your belly button in toward your spine.

- Work for up to one minute of deep breathing and ab toning.

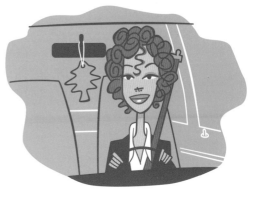

One minute of sitting actively burns 2 calories.
One minute of sitting while doing nothing else burns 1.1 calories.

ONE YEAR

2 calories x 5 days per week = 10 calories

10 calories x 50 weeks per year = 500 calories

500 calories ÷ 3,500 calories per pound = .14 pound

By sitting actively for one minute per day, you can burn off a little more than 1/8 pound per year.

5. on-the-road-again shoulder shrugs and circles

Traffic causes tension; it's unavoidable. Many people store tension in the neck and shoulder area. Loosen up tight shoulders with these shoulder shrugs and circles. Combining regular stretching and strengthening exercises and paying attention to good posture will relieve chronic tightness in these muscles.

> Sit upright with your shoulders relaxed and your hands on the steering wheel. (You can do this exercise while standing on the bus.)

> Exhale as you lift your shoulders up toward your ears, squeezing the muscles in your upper back, neck, and shoulders. Inhale as you hold the position.

> Exhale as you lower your shoulders, relaxing your muscles.

> Roll your shoulders up, back, down, and around, making shoulder circles and releasing muscular tension.

> Work for up to thirty seconds. Repeat again on the way home or during the day.

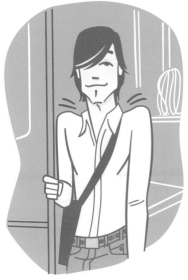

One minute of stretching burns 3.2 calories.
One minute of sitting while doing nothing else burns 1.1 calories.

ONE YEAR

3.2 calories x 5 days per week = 16 calories

16 calories x 50 weeks per year = 800 calories

800 calories ÷ 3,500 calories per pound = .23 pound

By adding one minute of shoulder shrugs and circles per day during your commute,
you can burn off almost 1/4 pound per year.

6. subway-flirting neck stretch

Take advantage of riding the subway to enjoy a neck stretch. Peer surreptitiously at your fellow commuters. Wink and smile at anyone interesting.

> Sit upright in your seat or stand with your shoulders relaxed and your arms at your sides.

> Inhale for four to five seconds.

> Exhale for five to six seconds as you turn your head to one side, feeling the stretch in your neck.

> Inhale deeply as you hold the stretch; exhale and see if you can turn your neck a bit farther to the side. Inhale as you return your head to center. Repeat one more time on the same side.

> Repeat the stretch on the other side.

Move through a comfortable range of motion. Keep arms
relaxed at your sides and your torso parallel to your seat back.

One minute of stretching burns 3.2 calories.
One minute of sitting while doing nothing else burns 1.1 calories.

ONE YEAR

3.2 calories x 5 days per week = 16 calories

16 calories x 50 weeks per year = 800 calories

800 calories ÷ 3,500 calories per pound = .23 pound

By adding one minute of commuting stretches per day, you can burn off almost
$1/4$ pound per year.

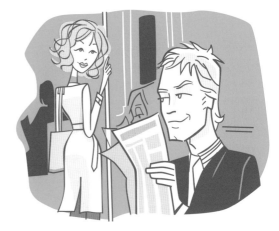

7. "get off my bumper" neck rolls

Sitting in traffic in front of someone who insists on hugging your car's bumper? Relieve neck tension with these neck rolls and encourage this commuter to get off your back as he wonders what you're doing.

> Sit upright in your seat with your shoulders relaxed and your hands in your lap.

> Inhale for four to five seconds.

> Exhale for five to six seconds as you tilt your head to one side, feeling the stretch in the side of your neck.

> Inhale.

> Exhale as you drop your chin to your chest and roll your opposite ear to your shoulder. Hold the head tilt to the side as you breathe deeply. Lift your head.

> Repeat the stretch on both sides.

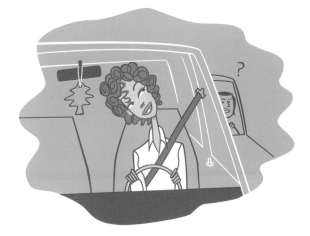

Move through a comfortable range of motion. Keep your arms relaxed at your sides and your toes parallel to the dashboard. Visualize tension draining from your neck and shoulders with each exhalation.

One minute of stretching burns 3.2 calories.
One minute of sitting while doing nothing else burns 1.1 calories.

ONE YEAR

3.2 calories x 5 days per week = 16 calories

16 calories x 50 weeks per year = 800 calories

800 calories ÷ 3,500 calories per pound = .23 pound

By adding one minute of commuting stretches per day, you can burn off almost 1/4 pound per year.

8. red-light forearm and wrist stretch

Zap tension in wrists and forearms while you're waiting for the signal to change. Soon you'll actually hope for road repair delays.

> Sit upright behind the wheel with your shoulders relaxed and your arms at your sides.

> Bend your left elbow so that your forearm is parallel to your lap.

> Flex your wrist and point your fingertips upward, palm facing forward.

> Place your right hand on your left palm.

> Inhale for four to five seconds.

> Exhale for five to six seconds as you gently press your left palm toward you, feeling the stretch on the bottom of your wrist and forearm.

> Inhale.

> Exhale as you bend your wrist and point your fingertips downward, palm facing your torso.

- Place your right hand on the back of your left hand.

- Inhale for four to five seconds.

- Exhale for five to six seconds as you gently press toward you on the back of your right hand, feeling the stretch on the top of your wrist and forearm.

- Repeat the stretches on the right arm.

SECRETS OF SUCCESS

Use gentle pressure. Breathe deeply. Keep your shoulders relaxed This is a particularly beneficial stretch if you work at a computer.

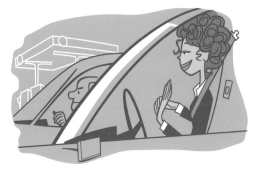

One minute of stretching burns 3.2 calories.
One minute of sitting while doing nothing else burns 1.1 calories.

ONE YEAR

3.2 calories x 5 days per week = 16 calories

16 calories x 50 weeks per year = 800 calories

800 calories ÷ 3,500 calories per pound = .23 pound

By adding one minute of commuting stretches per day, you can burn off almost ¹/₄ pound per year.

9. performance-maximizing parking lot stroll

Most people waste precious minutes circling the parking lot like hawks, seeking the spot closest to the entrance. Park quickly in the farthest spot and use those few extra minutes and the extra distance for a parking lot stroll. Your bottom line will improve.

> Stand with good posture.

> Pull your abdominal muscles in slightly to support your lower back.

> Look forward as you keep your head and chin level and your shoulders relaxed.

> Swing your arms naturally at your sides with your palms facing in.

> Walk at a gentle pace so that you can talk easily.

> Maintain an easy pace, slower than a twenty-minute mile.

> If you want to work harder, increase your pace.

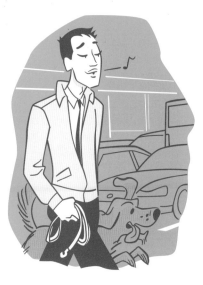

SECRETS OF SUCCESS

If rain keeps you from walking outside, invest in a good rain hat and coat or waterproof outerwear, so that weather will not prevent you from enjoying your daily stroll. Take advantage of casual Fridays. Studies show that when people wear more-casual clothes to the office, they move more and burn more calories.

One minute of strolling burns 3.8 calories.
One minute of standing burns 2 calories.

ONE YEAR

3.8 calories x 5 days per week = 19 calories
19 calories x 50 weeks per year = 950 calories
950 calories ÷ 3,500 calories per pound = .27 pound

By adding four minutes of walking per day to your daily routine, you can burn off more than 1 pound per year.

10. reach-for-the-top stair-climbing lunges

Stairwells are your friend. If your stairwell is dull, visualize yourself journeying up a steep trail loaded with your essential supplies for survival. Or imagine yourself climbing up the corporate ladder. Persevere—you will make it to the top.

> Stand upright, hold in your abdominal muscles, and relax your shoulders.

> Place your entire right foot on the second step above you.

> Push down on the step, lifting yourself up, feeling your buttocks and thighs contract.

> Place your entire left foot on the second step above your right foot.

> Continue to walk up, two steps at a time.

> Work for up to one minute.

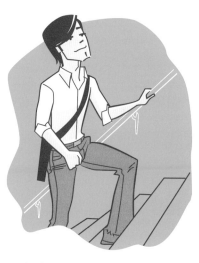

One minute of stair-climbing lunges burns 18 calories.
Riding the elevator burns 2 calories.

ONE YEAR

18 calories x 5 days per week = 90 calories

90 calories x 50 weeks per year = 4,500 calories

4,500 calories ÷ 3,500 calories per pound = 1.29 pounds

By adding one minute of stair-climbing per day at the office, instead of riding the elevator,
you can burn off almost 1 ¹/₃ pounds per year.

11. "i'm not quite ready to work!" chair squats

Before you take a seat and begin your day, practice lowering and lifting your tushie to tone your buttocks, hips, and thighs. Getting up and sitting down is one of the most important activities of daily life. The leading predictor of whether you will need assisted living in your old age is your leg strength. Do squats regularly not only for a toned backside, but also to maintain your physical independence as you age.

> Stand upright with your feet hip-width apart, about one inch in front of your chair. Hold in your abdominals and relax your shoulders.

> Inhale as you sit back, as if you are going to sit in your chair. Let your bottom lightly touch the chair without sitting down.

> Exhale as you push yourself back up to standing, while squeezing your buttocks.

> Work for up to one minute.

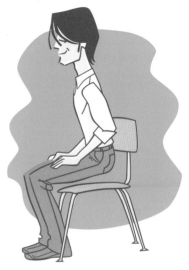

One minute of squats burns 10 calories.
One minute of sitting while doing nothing else burns 1.1 calories.

ONE YEAR

10 calories x 5 days per week = 50 calories
50 calories x 50 weeks per year = 2,500 calories
2,500 calories ÷ 3,500 calories per pound = .71 pound

By adding one minute of chair squats per day at the office, you can burn off almost ³/₄ pound per year.

12. ab-solutely wonderful work!
seated posture check and toner

Tone your abs while you sit in your chair, working hard. Listen for all the compliments on your stunning posture—and your well-done project.

> Sit in your chair on your sitz bones with your legs at a right angle and space behind your knees.

> Rest your feet on the ground hip-width apart. If your feet don't reach the floor, get a footrest.

> Draw your abdominal muscles in to support your lower back and keep your pelvis level.

> Lift your breastbone upward as you draw your lower rib cage in. Align your shoulders above your hips.

> Relax your shoulders. Allow your arms to hang at your sides.

> Lengthen the back of your neck, drawing your nose inward. Align your ears above your shoulders and keep your chin level.

> Inhale deeply, keeping your shoulders low and relaxed.

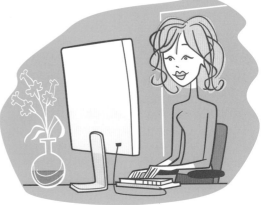

» Exhale completely, drawing your belly button toward your spine. Continue breathing deeply, using your abdominal muscles to assist the exhalation.

» Work for up to one minute.

One minute of sitting actively burns 2 calories, while sitting doing nothing else burns 1.1 calories. The main benefit of this exercise is toning and improved posture, which can prevent aches and pains, especially in the back.

ONE YEAR

2 calories x 5 days per week = 10 calories

10 calories x 50 weeks per year = 500 calories

500 calories ÷ 3,500 calories per pound = .14 pound

By sitting actively for one minute per day, you can burn off a little more than 1/8 pound per year and tone up your abs. You'll also improve your posture and reduce the likelihood of back pain.

13. "say no to aches and pains" desk and computer setup check

Good posture is key to achieving exercise results, preventing injuries, and keeping you pain-free over the years. Before performing any seated exercises, check your desk and computer setup. Movements you do repetitively have the greatest impact on your posture and well-being. One minute of abdominal crunches cannot undo the effects of eight hours of slouching. Set up your desk and computer properly to ensure that you are doing everything you can to support your body.

> Sit in your chair with good posture as described in Ab-solutely Wonderful Work! Seated Posture Check and Toner (page 36).

> Adjust your chair to fit your body. Set the seat height so your feet rest flat on the floor, with your knees bent approximately 90 degrees. If you cannot lower your seat enough, use a footrest to support your feet.

> Adjust the chair back to support the curve in your lower back. When you sit back in the chair, make sure you have at least an inch of space behind your knees so you do not compress your legs against the chair. If the seat is too deep, use a cushion to provide support for your lower back.

> Adjust the computer monitor to reinforce ideal seated posture and to protect your eyes. Elevate the top of the monitor to eye level with your head held straight. Place it one arm's length away, approximately sixteen to twenty-eight inches.

- Protect your wrists, neck, shoulders, and back with proper keyboard placement. Your keyboard should be parallel to your forearms or tilted slightly lower with your upper arms hanging at your sides. Avoid pressure on your wrists and keep your wrist joints in a neutral position with your wrists flat.

- If you use a mouse, keep it close to your keyboard so that you do not need to overreach to use it.

- Concentrate on maintaining your good seated posture throughout your workday. Be sure to get up often to move and stretch, at least a few minutes every hour.

- Studies show that getting up frequently lowers the risk of back pain.

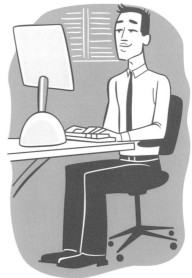

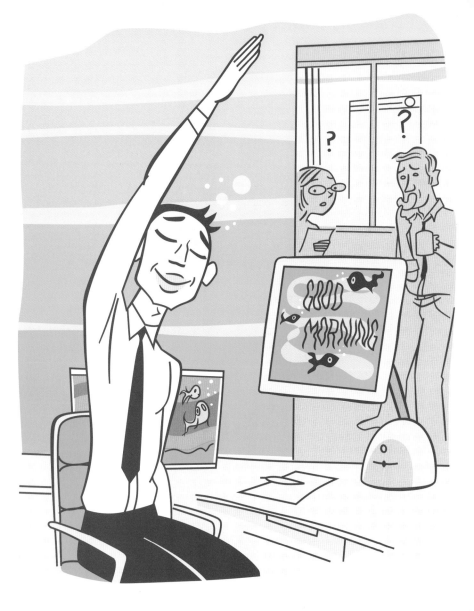

morning starters

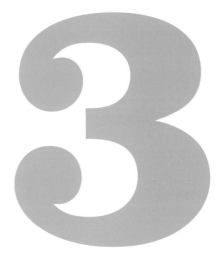

14. set-a-goal standing posture check

Stand upright, confident, and proud. Good posture prevents back pain and makes you appear slimmer and taller—some estimate as much as five pounds slimmer and one inch taller. Start the day off right and make good posture your goal. Whenever you stand, do a quick posture check. Use every opportunity to stand—while taking calls, organizing files, and, of course, checking your mail. Concentrate on posture as you stand and walk around. Remember, what you train is what you get! That is, if you frequently slouch, that's what you'll have when you look in the mirror. Every time you move is an opportunity to train your body for better posture.

> Stand with feet hip-width apart and the center of each foot parallel.

> Distribute your weight evenly on each foot. Lengthen behind your knees. Align your knees above your ankles.

> Draw your abdominal muscles inward. Keep your pelvis level and align your hips above your knees.

> Lift your breastbone upward as you draw your lower rib cage inward. Align your shoulders above your hips.

> Relax your shoulders. Allow your arms to hang at your sides with palms in.

> Lengthen the back of your neck, drawing your nose inward. Align your ears above your shoulders.

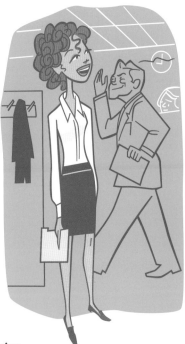

One minute of standing burns 2 calories.
One minute of sitting while doing nothing else burns 1.1 calories.

ONE YEAR

2 calories x 5 days per week = 10 calories

10 calories x 50 weeks per year = 500 calories

500 calories ÷ 3,500 calories per pound = .14 pound

By standing for one minute per day, instead of sitting, you can burn off almost 1/8 pound per year. Standing burns twice as many calories as sitting. Stand as often as possible to use more energy.

15. hit-a-home-run elbow butterflies stretch

Release tension in your neck and shoulders while you wait for your computer to get fired up. Start the day right by counteracting the tendency to collapse your chest while sitting at your desk. Greet the day feeling refreshed, open, and ready to make it happen.

> Sit with good posture.

> Place your fingertips on the back of your head, thumbs on the base of your skull.

> Inhale deeply as you hold your elbows out wide, squeezing your shoulder blades together and feeling a stretch in the front of your shoulders and chest.

> Exhale as you bring your elbows together in front of your nose, feeling a stretch in the backs of your shoulders and in your upper back.

> Continue to open and close your elbows as you breathe deeply, releasing tension in the upper back, chest, and shoulders. Continue for at least thirty seconds.

> To increase the upper back and neck stretch, drop your chin toward your chest as your elbows are in the forward position. Breathe deeply, releasing tension and stress with each exhalation as you hold the stretch for up to thirty seconds.

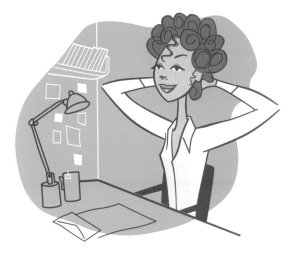

One minute of stretching burns 3.2 calories.
One minute of sitting while doing nothing else burns 1.1 calories.

ONE YEAR

3.2 calories x 5 days per week = 16 calories

16 calories x 50 weeks per year = 800 calories

800 calories ÷ 3,500 calories per pound = .23 pound

By adding one minute of desk stretches per day, you can burn off almost ¹/₄ pound
per year.

16. did you see that e-mail? chest stretch

As you read lengthy e-mails, use the time to stretch your chest and shoulders. This stretch is particularly valuable to counteract rounded shoulders from the tendency to slouch as you sit at your desk. The more aware you become of your posture during the workday, the less you will slouch.

> Sit with good posture with your shoulders relaxed, arms at your sides and palms facing in.

> Clasp your hands together behind your lower back. Keep your abdominal muscles tight to support your lower back.

> Inhale.

> Exhale as you squeeze your shoulder blades together and gently lift your hands to stretch your upper chest and the front of your shoulders.

> Inhale as you hold the stretch.

> Exhale as you gently try to increase the stretch by further lifting your clasped hands.

> Breathe deeply as you hold the stretch for at least thirty seconds. Repeat, if desired.

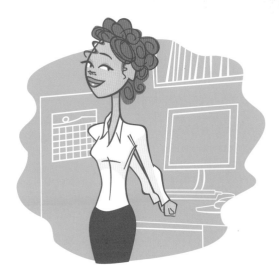

Avoid arching your lower back. Stretch only to the point
of moderate tension, moving gently and deliberately.
Increase the stretch by trying to bring your palms together.

One minute of stretching burns 3.2 calories.
One minute of sitting while doing nothing else burns 1.1 calories.

ONE YEAR
3.2 calories x 5 days per week = 16 calories
16 calories x 50 weeks per year = 800 calories
800 calories ÷ 3,500 calories per pound = .23 pound

By stretching for one minute per day at your desk, you can burn off almost 1/4 pound
per year.

17. sit-up-and-succeed chest and shoulder opener

Lengthen your posture with this energizing stretch that counteracts the tendency to slouch. You will feel better and project a more confident image. Confidence in the office is always great, especially when asking for your well-deserved raise.

> Sit with good posture with your shoulders relaxed and your arms at your sides.

> Spread your arms out wide as you reach toward opposite sides of the room. Rotate your palms upward and lift your arms overhead. Stretch your fingertips as if you want to touch the sky.

> Gently clasp your hands together. Inhale as you arch your upper back and lift your breastbone upward. Exhale as you hold the stretch.

> Continue to breathe deeply as you stretch and lengthen your torso for up to thirty seconds.

> For an additional back stretch, lower your clasped hands in front of your chest. Breathe deeply as you relax your shoulders and spread your shoulder blades wide across your back.

> Repeat by reaching your arms wide, then lifting upward to continue stretching for another thirty seconds.

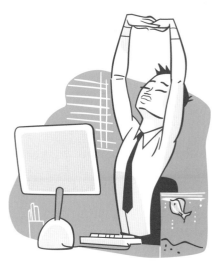

Feel your chest, back, and torso open and lengthen as you reach wide and then up. Breathe deeply and follow the flow of energy through your body as you stretch to the point of moderate tension. Release tightness as you exhale.

One minute of stretching burns 3.2 calories.
One minute of sitting while doing nothing else burns 1.1 calories.

ONE YEAR

3.2 calories x 5 days per week = 16 calories

16 calories x 50 weeks per year = 800 calories

800 calories ÷ 3,500 calories per pound = .23 pound

By stretching for one minute per day at your desk, you can burn off almost ¹/₄ pound per year.

18. "good morning!" side and wrist stretch

Greet your colleagues with a friendly and energizing wave as you sneak in a stretch that improves the health of your back and wrists. Keyboarding stresses your wrists. Waving warms up your wrists by lubricating the joints, thereby reducing your risk of wrist injury and helping you to feel great.

> Sit with good posture with your shoulders relaxed and your arms at your sides.

> Lift your left arm, palm up, in a long arc overhead until your palm faces down. Feel the stretch in the side of your torso.

> Continue stretching through the side of your torso as you move your wrist side to side as if you are waving to a colleague. This wrist movement warms up your wrist joint and improves wrist mobility.

> Continue to breathe deeply as you stretch and wave for up to thirty seconds.

> Repeat on the other side.

Avoid arching your lower back by keeping your
abdominal muscles pulled inward. Focus on lifting
upward and outward. Avoid collapsing into your waist.

One minute of stretching burns 3.2 calories.
One minute of sitting while doing nothing else burns 1.1 calories.

ONE YEAR

3.2 calories x 5 days per week = 16 calories

16 calories x 50 weeks per year = 800 calories

800 calories ÷ 3,500 calories per pound = .23 pound

By stretching one minute per day at your desk,
you can burn off almost $1/4$ pound per year.

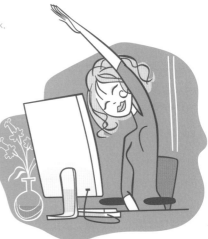

19. "who else is here this early?" seated spine twist

Check out who made it to the office as early as you did and enjoy a stretch for your lower back and hips that also lubricates the joints of your spine. Spinal rotation is an important movement—if you don't do it, you will lose the ability to turn at the waist. So take a look around the office and keep your back healthy.

- ❯ Sit with good posture with your shoulders relaxed and your arms at your sides.

- ❯ Keep your hips and feet facing your desk as you rotate your waist, ribs, and shoulders to the right and bring your left hand across your right thigh. Sit up tall, keeping length through your spine as you rotate your neck and look over your right shoulder.

- ❯ Inhale as you lengthen your spine, keeping your shoulders level. Exhale as you try to increase the stretch, using your left hand against your thigh for leverage. Breathe deeply as you hold the stretch for up to thirty seconds.

- ❯ Repeat on the other side.

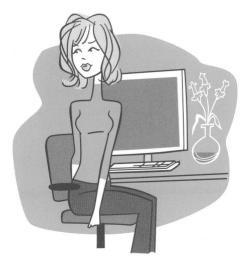

One minute of stretching burns 3.2 calories.
One minute of sitting while doing nothing else burns 1.1 calories.

ONE YEAR

3.2 calories x 5 days per week = 16 calories

16 calories x 50 weeks per year = 800 calories

800 calories ÷ 3,500 calories per pound = .23 pound

By stretching at your desk for one minute per day, you can burn off almost ¼ pound per year.

20. "what's on top of my filing cabinet?" one-legged squats

While you survey the forgotten coffee cups and misplaced phone messages on top of the filing cabinet, lower yourself down on one leg for a closer look. Use good technique to simultaneously tone your hips and thighs and improve your core muscles and balance. Try some one-legged squats while you're talking on the phone to really test your powers of concentration. Good balance prevents falls, and avoiding falls prevents injuries, including fatal accidents. Challenge your balance daily. It just might save your life.

> Stand upright, hold in your abdominals, and relax your shoulders.

> Place your right hand on a filing cabinet, chair, desk, or wall for support.

> Stand on your right leg as you lift your left thigh and bend your knee. Squeeze your right hip to stabilize yourself.

> Inhale as you bend your right knee and lower your hips as if you are going to sit in a chair.

> Exhale as you return to standing position.

> Continue for eight to twelve repetitions or for thirty seconds.

> Repeat with the other leg.

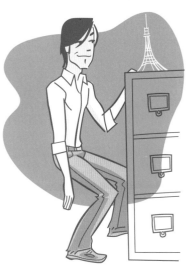

VARIATION

To make the squats a little more
challenging, try not using the cabinet
for balance.

SECRETS OF SUCCESS

Use your core muscles and tighten your abdominals to keep
your posture strong. Avoid dropping your head forward.
Lengthen the back of your neck to keep your ears above
your shoulders. Keep your knee over your foot.

One minute of one-legged squats burns 10 calories.
One minute of sitting while doing nothing else burns 1.1 calories.

ONE YEAR

10 calories x 5 days per week = 50 calories
50 calories x 50 weeks per year = 2,500 calories
2,500 calories ÷ 3,500 calories per pound = .71 pound

By adding one minute of squats per day, instead of simply standing in your cubicle, you
can burn off a little more than ²/₃ pound per year and tone up your hips and thighs.

21. "hand me a thumbtack!" triceps hammers

Prevent underarm jiggle while your co-workers think you're redecorating your cubicle with inspirational posters. Keeping your triceps strong enables you to push open heavy doors, push yourself up from armchairs, and hammer nails. Fill up your water bottle for an instant portable weight.

> Stand in front of a wall with a weighted water bottle in your right hand.

> Take a generous step back with your right foot and keep your weight on the ball of your foot. Keep your abdominal muscles tight to support your lower back.

> Raise your right arm to shoulder height and bend your elbow, lowering the weighted hand toward your right shoulder.

> Exhale as you straighten your right arm as if you are hammering a nail into the wall.

> Continue for eight to twelve repetitions or for thirty seconds.

> Switch sides and repeat.

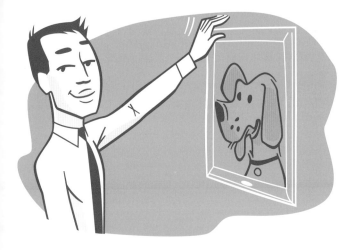

One minute of triceps hammers burns 10 calories.
One minute of standing burns 2 calories.

ONE YEAR

10 calories x 5 days per week = 50 calories

50 calories x 50 weeks per year = 2,500 calories

2,500 calories ÷ 3,500 calories per pound = .71 pound

By adding one minute of triceps hammers per day instead of standing in your cubicle, you
can burn off a little more than $^2/_3$ pound per year and tone up your hips and thighs.

22. "good morning, neighbor!" office walk

When you're ready to get your morning coffee, use the time to take a large lap around the office, greet your co-workers, and enjoy an energizing walk. Just be sure to avoid Wanda in accounting who brought in those cinnamon buns!

- Stand with good posture.

- Pull your abdominals in slightly to support your lower back.

- Look forward as you keep your head and chin level and your shoulders relaxed.

- Bend your elbows 90 degrees and hold your hands in relaxed fists with your palms facing in and your arms swinging rhythmically.

- Walk at a moderate pace so that you can greet your co-workers.

- Keep moving like you're eager to start your day. Break a light sweat.

- Maintain a twenty-minute-mile pace.

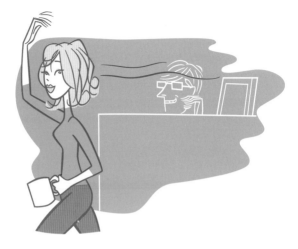

SECRETS OF SUCCESS

Hold an empty mug in one hand so that when you pump your arms, it will look like you're doing it because you're carrying your mug. Walk to another floor to add even more distance and an extra stair climb.

One minute of walking at a three-mile-per-hour pace burns 4.2 calories.
One minute of standing burns 2 calories.

ONE YEAR

4.2 calories x 5 days per week = 21 calories
21 calories x 50 weeks per year = 1,050 calories
1,050 calories ÷ 3,500 calories per pound = .3 pound

By adding three minutes of walking per day, you can burn off up to 1 pound per year.

23. early-bird coffeepot curls

Before you pour your morning cup of coffee, add a few lifts with the coffeepot. Your biceps will benefit from the extra toning. For a real challenge, beat your co-workers to the pot so that you can lift it when it's brimming full and at its heaviest. Enjoy the rewards of your labor as you sip your very fresh coffee.

> Stand with good posture, holding the coffeepot with your right hand.

> Inhale as you straighten your right arm, lowering the coffeepot as low as possible without spilling. Keep your wrist neutral and your elbow close to your waist.

> Exhale as you bend your right elbow and lift the coffeepot up toward your right shoulder.

> Continue for eight to twelve repetitions or for thirty seconds.

> Switch sides and repeat.

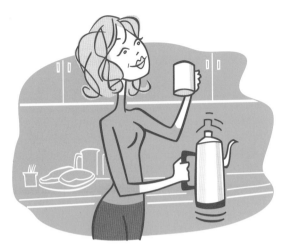

One minute of coffeepot curls burns 10 calories.
One minute of standing burns 2 calories.

ONE YEAR
10 calories x 5 days per week = 50 calories
50 calories x 50 weeks per year = 2,500 calories
2,500 calories ÷ 3,500 calories per pound = .71 pound

By adding one minute of coffeepot curls per day instead of simply standing, you can burn
off a little more than ½ pound per year and tone up your arms.

24. keeping-your-eyes-on-the-prize standing back extension

Focus on your goals—or just check out what's on the ceiling—while you give your back some needed relief. This stretch relieves stiffness from sitting for long periods of time and helps to maintain a healthy curve in your lower spine. It also counteracts the negative effects of slouching. Just say no to rounded shoulders and a collapsed chest.

» Stand with your feet hip-width apart. Place your hands on your lower back.

» Inhale slowly as you gently arch your lower back, using your hands for support. Take your head back only as far as you are comfortable. Avoid arching your neck too far back.

» Exhale while returning to an upright position as you draw your abdominal muscles inward to support your back.

» Repeat three to six times as comfortable.

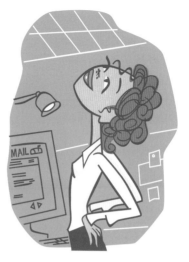

One minute of stretching burns 3.2 calories.
One minute of sitting while doing nothing else burns 1.1 calories.

ONE YEAR

3.2 calories x 5 days per week = 16 calories

16 calories x 50 weeks per year = 800 calories

800 calories ÷ 3,500 calories per pound = .23 pound

By standing and stretching your torso for one minute per day, instead of sitting, you can
burn off almost $\frac{1}{4}$ pound per year. Keeping your spine flexible helps you to maintain a
healthy back and to avoid aches and pains.

25. no-limits stairwell bun-blaster

Deliver interoffice messages in person. Your office building's stairwell is the next best thing to a piece of cardio equipment. Climbing stairs burns almost ten times more calories than taking the elevator. Tone up your buttocks and legs, get your heart pumping, and energize yourself.

> Stand upright, hold in your abdominal muscles, and relax your shoulders.

> Place your entire right foot on the step.

> Push down on the step, lifting yourself up, feeling your buttocks and thighs contract. Continue climbing the stairs in this fashion.

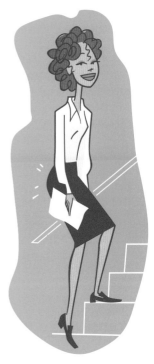

VARIATION

For more of a challenge, turn the stairwell into your private weight training *and* cardio studio. Tone up your hips and thighs by adding Reach for the Top Stair-climbing Lunges (page 32) to your bun-blasting cardio climbs. For example, climb one flight of stairs one step at a time. Climb the next flight two steps at a time. Keep alternating as long as time and your energy permit.

SECRETS OF SUCCESS

Start with one flight of stairs. Take the elevator to one flight below your destination. Walk up to your floor. Increase the number of flights as you become fitter.

**One minute of stair-climbing burns 18 calories.
Riding the elevator burns about 2 calories.**

ONE YEAR

18 calories x 5 calories days per week = 90 calories

90 calories x 50 weeks per year = 4,500 calories

4,500 calories ÷ 3,500 calories per pound = 1.29 pounds

By adding one minute of stair-climbing per day at the office, you can burn off almost 1 1/3 pounds per year.

26. "prairie dog" cubicle calf raises

Pop your head above the old cubicle wall and check out what's going on around the office. It's a great way to tone your legs, and standing in your cubicle provides the perfect chance to give yourself a lift. This is also a great exercise to do while you're on the phone.

- ❯ Stand upright, hold in your abdominal muscles, and relax your shoulders.

- ❯ Place one hand on a chair, desk, filing cabinet, or wall for support.

- ❯ Stand on one leg. Exhale as you push up onto the ball of your foot, lifting your body weight on the standing leg.

- ❯ Inhale as you lower your heel toward the floor without resting completely.

- ❯ Continue for thirty seconds.

- ❯ Switch legs and repeat.

VARIATION

Get started with an easier version by lifting and lowering with both feet. As you grow stronger, progress to lifting up with both feet and lowering only on one. Increase the difficulty when the exercise becomes easy to perform by not holding anything for support. This challenges your core muscles to keep your balance while you are strengthening your leg muscles.

SECRETS OF SUCCESS

Lift high to fully contract the calf muscle. Pay attention to the level of difficulty. When you notice that an exercise is becoming easier, change to a more difficult variation. This way, you won't get bored and you'll keep getting stronger.

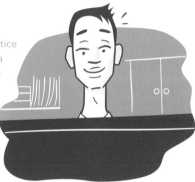

One minute of calf raises burns 10 calories.
One minute of standing burns 2 calories.

ONE YEAR

10 calories x 5 days per week = 50 calories
50 calories x 50 weeks per year = 2,500 calories
2,500 calories ÷ 3,500 calories per pound = .71 pound

By adding one minute of calf raises per day, instead of simply standing in your cubicle, you can burn off a little more than ²/₃ pound per year and tone up your calves.

27. "has anyone seen the mcclasky report?" standing calf stretch

Take every opportunity to stand. When searching for papers on your desk, stand, survey, and stretch out your calves. Keeping your calves flexible can prevent heel pain and a shuffling gait.

> Stand with your feet hip-width apart in front of your desk with your hips parallel to the desk and your shoulders relaxed.

> Place your hands on your desk, keeping good spinal alignment.

> Take one generous step backward with your right foot, keeping your foot pointing straight ahead.

> Push your heel into the ground, straightening your leg as much as you can.

> Breathe comfortably and feel the stretch in your lower leg. Hold for thirty seconds.

> Repeat on the other side.

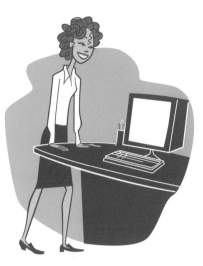

One minute of stretching burns 3.2 calories.
One minute of sitting while doing nothing else burns 1.1 calories.

ONE YEAR

3.2 calories x 5 days per week = 16 calories

16 calories x 50 weeks per year = 800 calories

800 calories ÷ 3,500 calories per pound = .23 pound

By standing and stretching your calves for one minute per day, instead of sitting, you can burn off almost ¼ pound per year.

28. waiting-for-that-fax push-ups

Working in an office makes it difficult to build and keep upper body strength. Add some wall push-ups to your day while you wait for a fax or the photocopier. Tone up your chest, back, arms, shoulders, and abdominal muscles for a minimal investment of your time.

> Stand hip-width apart, facing a stable wall.

> Place your hands on the wall slightly below shoulder level and slightly wider than shoulder-width apart. Tighten your abdominals to support your back.

> Inhale as you bend your elbows and lower your chest and torso, keeping good spinal alignment. Avoid dropping your head.

> Exhale as you push up to the starting position.

> Do eight to twelve repetitions or work for up to one minute.

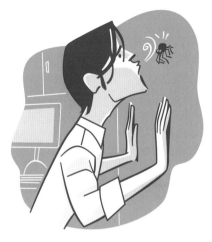

VARIATION

For more of a challenge, place your hands on the edge
of a desk and do the exercise as described.

SECRETS OF SUCCESS

Do not do this exercise if you experience wrist pain.
Strengthen your forearms first with wrist exercises
(page 74) and reverse curls (page 16).

**One minute of push-ups burns 10 calories.
One minute of standing burns 2 calories.**

ONE YEAR

10 calories x 5 days per week = 50 calories
50 calories x 50 weeks per year = 2,500 calories
2,500 calories ÷ 3,500 calories per pound = .71 pound

By adding one minute of wall push-ups per day, instead of simply standing, you can burn
off almost ³/₄ pound per year and tone your upper body.

29. catching-up-on-gossip side raise

Do this exercise while wearing your headset and your co-workers will think you're having a very animated conversation. You can use an exercise band or a full water bottle for resistance to strengthen your shoulders. Toned shoulders reduce the risk of shoulder injuries and create a broader shoulder line, which contributes to a slimmer appearance.

> Sit comfortably in your chair, shoulders relaxed, arms at sides, holding a band in front of your body or a weighted water bottle in your right hand. Tighten your abdominal muscles to support your back. Maintain good posture (page 36).

> Exhale as you lift your right arm out to the side and up to shoulder height. Keep your shoulders relaxed, your torso stable, and your wrist flat.

> Inhale as you lower your arm to the starting position.

> Do eight to twelve repetitions or work for thirty seconds.

> Switch arms and repeat.

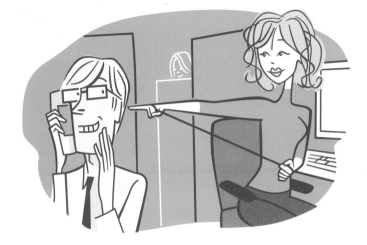

SECRETS OF SUCCESS
Do not do this exercise if you experience wrist pain.
Strengthen your forearms first with wrist exercises (page
74) and reverse curls (page 16). Keep your shoulders down,
your chest lifted, and your abs tight, maintaining good
posture throughout the exercise.

One minute of side raises burns 10 calories.
One minute of sitting while doing nothing else burns 1.1 calories.

ONE YEAR
10 calories x 5 days per week = 50 calories
50 calories x 50 weeks per year = 2,500 calories
2,500 calories ÷ 3,500 calories per pound = .71 pound

By adding one minute of side raises per day, instead of simply sitting at your desk, you can
burn off almost ³/₄ pound per year and tone up your shoulders.

30. power-keyboarding seated water-bottle wrist curls and extensions

Toned wrists may not get you noticed at the office Christmas party, but they will prevent wrist pain after working long hours on the keyboard. Use a water bottle filled to a weight that you can handle for this exercise. You'll notice a difference in your wrists and forearms after only a few short weeks of doing these lifts regularly.

WRIST EXTENSIONS

> Sit comfortably in your chair with your shoulders relaxed and holding a weighted water bottle in your right hand. Tighten your abdominal muscles to support your back.

> Place your right forearm on your right thigh, palm down, with your wrist joint extended beyond your knee.

> Exhale as you lift the back of your hand up toward your forearm, lifting the water bottle. Keep your shoulders relaxed.

> Inhale as you return to the starting position.

> Do eight to twelve repetitions or for thirty seconds.

> Repeat with left arm.

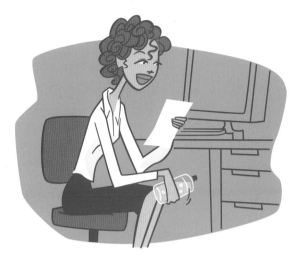

> Perform the previous exercise, but with your palm facing up.

SECRETS OF SUCCESS

Do not do this exercise if you experience wrist pain.

One minute of wrist curls and extensions burns 5 calories.
One minute of sitting while doing nothing else burns 1.1 calories.

ONE YEAR

5 calories x 5 days per week = 25 calories

25 calories x 50 weeks per year = 1,250 calories

1,250 calories ÷ 3,500 calories per pound = .35 pound

By adding two minutes of wrist exercises per day, instead of simply sitting at your desk, you can burn off almost ³/₄ pound per year and strengthen your wrists.

31. office-tour bathroom break

Get up periodically and give your body a break from sitting at your workstation. It's the best way to avoid aches and pains. When nature calls and you must tear yourself away from your desk, use the opportunity to take the long way to the restroom.

> Stand with good posture.

> Pull your abdominals in slightly to support your lower back.

> Look forward as you keep your head and chin level and your shoulders relaxed.

> Bend your elbows 90 degrees and hold your hands in relaxed fists with your palms facing in and your arms swinging rhythmically.

> Walk at a moderate pace and enjoy an office tour.

> Keep moving like you're eager to get back to work. Break a light sweat.

> Maintain a twenty-minute-mile pace.

> Walk faster to use more energy.

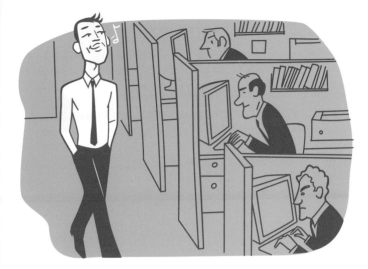

Carry a large manila envelope or file folder in your hands and walk as if you're late for a meeting. No one will even raise an eyebrow over the fact that you're traveling so briskly down the hall!

One minute of walking at a three-mile-per-hour pace burns 4.2 calories.
One minute of standing burns 2 calories.

ONE YEAR

4.2 calories x 5 days per week = 21 calories
21 calories x 50 weeks per year = 1,050 calories
1,050 calories ÷ 3,500 calories per pound = .3 pound

By adding three minutes of walking to your daily routine, you can burn off up to 1 pound per year.

32. top-secret-meeting triceps push-ups

Enjoy a little private time in the restroom. Use an available wall to work triceps toning into your day. No one needs to know your secrets.

> Stand hip-width apart, facing a stable wall.

> Place your hands on the wall just below shoulder level in a diamond or triangular shape. Tighten your abdominals to support your back.

> Inhale as you bend your elbows and lower your chest and torso, keeping good spinal alignment. Avoid dropping your head.

> Exhale as you push up to the starting position.

> Do eight to twelve repetitions or work for up to one minute.

VARIATIONS

Instead of using the wall, do your push-ups with your hands on the edge of the sink for more of a challenge. Since your body is at more of an angle, your muscles need to work harder to lift your body weight against gravity. You can also do sink push-ups in the morning or evening immediately after you brush your teeth.

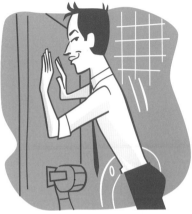

SECRETS OF SUCCESS

Do not do this exercise if you experience wrist pain. Strengthen your forearms first with wrist exercises (page 74) and reverse curls (page 16).

One minute of triceps push-ups burns 10 calories.
One minute of standing burns 2 calories.

ONE YEAR

10 calories x 5 days per week = 50 calories
50 calories x 50 weeks per year = 2,500 calories
2,500 calories ÷ 3,500 calories per pound = .71 pound

By adding one minute of wall or sink push-ups per day, instead of simply standing in the restroom, you can burn off almost ³/₄ pound per year and tone up the backs of your arms.

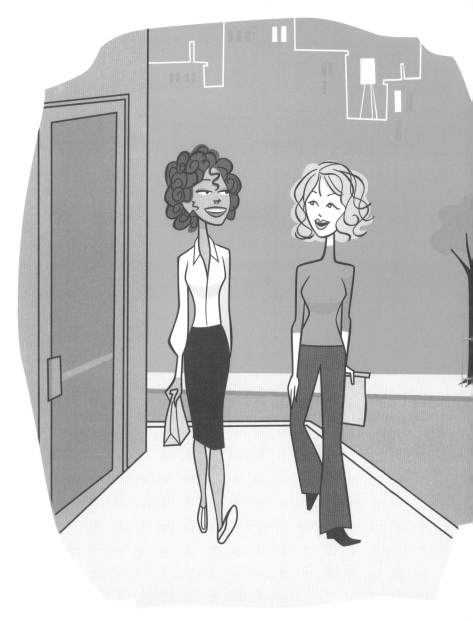

lunchtime energizers

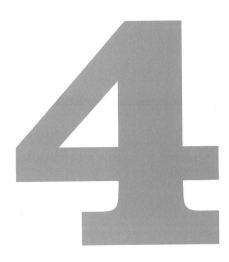

33. play-to-win lunch fitness walk

Fitting in exercise during your lunch hour breaks up your day and clears your mind for a productive afternoon. At day's end, family responsibilities and fatigue can get in the way of your best intentions. Use your lunchtime to be sure you get in a workday workout. Be sure to wear supportive athletic shoes and comfortable, breathable clothes. Invest in two pairs of athletic shoes, so you can always leave one pair at the office.

» Start strolling with good posture, arms swinging rhythmically at your sides (page 58).

» As you start feeling more warmed-up, bend your elbows 90 degrees, hold your hands in relaxed fists, and continue swinging your arms rhythmically as you increase to a moderate pace. This pace equals three miles per hour, about 105 steps per minute.

» To increase intensity, increase to a moderate-to-brisk pace, so you can still talk but not easily carry on a conversation. This pace equals four miles per hour, about 140 steps per minute. Continue for at least ten minutes.

» For the last eight minutes of your walk, slow to a moderate pace and then to a stroll before you finish.

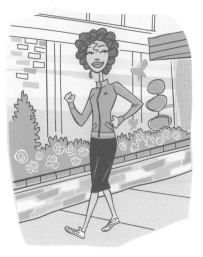

**One minute of walking at a pace of four miles per hour
burns 6 calories.**
One minute of standing burns 2 calories.

ONE YEAR
6 calories x 5 days per week = 30 calories
30 calories x 50 weeks per year = 1,500 calories
1,500 calories ÷ 3,500 calories per pound = .42 pounds

By adding ten minutes of moderate-to-brisk walking to your workday routine per day, you
can burn off a little more than 4 1/4 pounds per year.

34. power-lunch fitness walk II: timed intervals

Vary your walking pace for measured increments to add variety and to improve your conditioning level by working at higher intensities for short periods of times. Intervals are organized by time or by distance. This workout equals twenty-eight minutes.

> Warm up for five minutes with an easy stroll (page 30), at a pace of less than three miles per hour.

> Increase your intensity to a moderate pace (page 58) for five minutes. This pace equals three miles per hour, about 105 steps per minute.

> Increase your intensity to a moderate-to-brisk-paced fitness walk (page 82) for one minute. This pace equals four miles per hour, about 140 steps per minute.

> Reduce your intensity to a moderately paced walk for five minutes.

> Repeat the fitness walk for one minute.

> Reduce your intensity to a moderately paced walk for five minutes.

> Repeat the fitness walk for one minute.

> Cool down with an easy stroll for five minutes.

Adjust the intensity to correspond with your energy level.
If you want to increase intensity, shorten the moderately
paced intervals (page 58) and increase the fitness walk
intervals (page 82). If you want to reduce intensity,
eliminate the fitness walk intervals and alternate between
an easy stroll (page 30) and moderate walk (page 58).

**One minute of easy strolling at less than three miles per hour burns
3.8 calories.**
**One minute of moderately paced walking at a three-mile-per-hour
pace burns 4 calories.**
**One minute of fitness walking at a four-mile-per-hour pace burns
6 calories.**
One minute of standing burns 2 calories.

ONE YEAR

3.8 calories x 10 minutes = 38 calories

4 calories x 15 minutes = 60 calories

6 calories x 3 minutes = 18 calories

116 calories x 1 day per week = 116 calories

116 calories x 50 weeks per year = 5,800 calories

5,800 calories ÷ 3,500 calories per pound = 1.66 pounds

By adding one timed interval walk to your weekly routine, you can burn off up to
1 2/3 pounds per year.

35. strength-lunch fitness walk III: toning circuit

Mix toning exercises with your lunchtime walk for a combination workout that achieves more results in less time. This workout burns energy, conditions your heart and lungs, and tones your upper and lower body in a total of forty minutes.

> Warm up for five minutes with an easy stroll (page 30), at a pace of less than three miles per hour.

> Increase your intensity to a moderate pace (page 58) or a moderate-to-brisk fitness pace (page 82) for five minutes.

> Do squats (page 34) for about one minute.

> Resume a moderately paced walk or fitness walk for ten minutes.

> Do push-ups (page 70) against a wall, tree, or bench for one minute.

> Resume a moderately paced walk or fitness walk for ten minutes.

> Do alternating lunges (page 32) for one minute. Step forward onto a stair or onto the ground in front of you. Push yourself back up to the starting position. Step forward with the other leg. Continue alternating for one minute. Since you're not lifting your body weight up the stairs, the caloric count for these lunges is lower and similar to other toning exercises.

> Cool down with an easy stroll for five minutes.

> Do thirty seconds of reverse curls (page 16).

(page 16)

SECRETS OF SUCCESS

Incorporate other toning exercises during the one-minute toning segments for variety. Use your resistance band or weighted water bottle for toning exercises as needed. To make it easy to carry, tie the band around your waist. Hold your water bottle in your hand or purchase a waist pack that has a water-bottle carrier. Whenever you use equipment, avoid gripping it tightly; instead, use a steady but relaxed grip. Avoid white knuckles and breath holding, as they can raise your blood pressure. Breathe deeply, let go of stress, and enjoy your walk.

One minute of circuit training burns approximately 6 calories. One minute of standing burns 2 calories.

. . . .

ONE YEAR

6 calories x 40 minutes = 240 calories
240 calories x 1 day per week = 240 calories
240 calories x 50 weeks per year = 12,000 calories
12,000 calories ÷ 3,500 calories per pound = 3.43 pounds

By adding one toning circuit walk to your weekly routine, you can burn off up to 3 1/2 pounds per year.

36. number-crunching shoulder-blade squeezes with band

After a morning of crunching the numbers and squeezing profit out of your budget, midday is an ideal time to squeeze your shoulders. Sitting for hours at a desk can lead to rounded shoulders and a slouchy posture. This toner strengthens your back muscles and lifts and opens your chest and shoulders. Stronger back muscles reduce chronic neck and shoulder tension. Use an exercise band for resistance as described below. Keep your band at the office on your desk or in a top desk drawer as a reminder to fit in your exercises.

➤ Sit comfortably in your chair or stand, shoulders relaxed, arms at sides, holding a band in front of your body in both hands. Tighten your abdominals to support your back. Maintain good posture (page 36).

➤ Exhale as you squeeze your shoulder blades together. Keep your shoulders relaxed, torso stable, and wrists flat.

➤ Inhale as you return your arm to the starting position.

➤ Do eight to twelve repetitions or work for up to one minute.

➤ Rest and repeat.

Keep your chest open and lifted. Avoid arching your lower back or hunching your shoulders. Strengthening these muscles leads to improved posture and a more confident and relaxed appearance. Do not perform this exercise if you have any pain or discomfort in your shoulders.

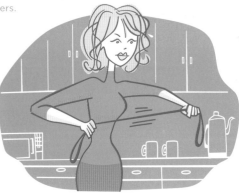

One minute of shoulder-blade squeezes burns 10 calories.
One minute of sitting while doing nothing else burns 1.1 calories.

ONE YEAR

10 calories x 5 days per week = 50 calories

50 calories x 50 weeks per year = 2,500 calories

2,500 calories ÷ 3,500 calories per pound = .71 pound

By adding one minute of shoulder-blade squeezes per day, instead of simply sitting at your desk, you can burn off almost ¾ pound per year and tone up your shoulders.

37. climbing-the-corporate-ladder lat pull-downs with band

Improve your posture and tone up the sides of your torso under your arms with this great exercise that works your "climbing" muscles, known formally as your latissimus dorsi, or lats. We need to challenge these muscles, since our lifestyle today, unlike the lives of cavemen, does not require us to use these muscles actively. Combat office slouch and tone these important postural muscles with a minimal investment of time and effort. As your back becomes stronger, you'll be amazed at how much taller you stand and how much better you feel. Use your handy exercise band for resistance.

> Sit comfortably in your chair or stand, holding the end of a resistance band in each hand. Lift your arms overhead without hunching your shoulders, palms facing front. Tighten your abdominals to support back. Maintain good posture (page 42).

> Keep your left arm elevated as you exhale and bend your right elbow, pulling your right hand down and lowering your right elbow down and back toward your waist. Keep your shoulders level and chest open.

> Inhale as you raise your right arm back up to the starting position.

> Do eight to twelve repetitions or work for up to thirty seconds.

> Repeat the exercise on the other side.

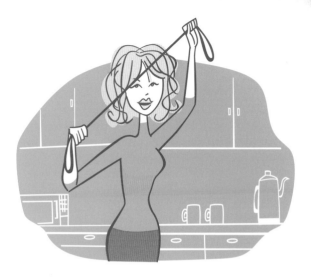

Imagine you are pulling yourself up a ladder or doing chin-ups with one arm. Visualize yourself successfully rising up the corporate ladder. Keep your chest open and lifted. Avoid arching your lower back. Feel the contraction on the side of your torso that is targeted by the exercise.

One minute of lat pull-downs burns 10 calories.
One minute of sitting while doing nothing else burns 1.1 calories.

ONE YEAR

10 calories x 5 days per week = 50 calories
50 calories x 50 weeks per year = 2,500 calories
2,500 calories ÷ 3,500 calories per pound = .71 pound

By adding one minute of lat pull-downs per day, instead of simply sitting at your desk, you can burn off almost ³/₄ pound per year and tone up your back and torso.

38. stretching-the-budget standing hamstring stretch

Take a standing break and keep your muscles flexible and your back healthy. Tight hamstrings can contribute to lower back pain. To get the best results, try to stretch daily, or at least two to three times per week. If you're feeling tighter than usual, make sure you are drinking plenty of water. Our muscles are 72 percent water, and even slight dehydration affects performance.

> Stand with your feet hip-width apart and your right foot less than one full step in front of your left foot.

> Exhale as you bend your hips and back knee as if you are sitting back, and lengthen your front leg, feeling the stretch in the back of your leg.

> Place your hand on the thigh of your bent leg for support, avoiding any pressure on the knee joint. Keep your abdominal muscles tight to support your lower back. Relax your shoulders and maintain neutral spinal alignment.

> Breathe normally as you hold the stretch for thirty seconds.

> Release the stretch, stand upright, and repeat on the other side.

Avoid collapsing your chest or rounding your shoulders forward. Lengthen your spine as you keep your shoulders relaxed and your abdominal muscles tightened.

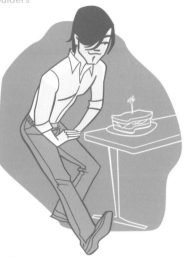

One minute of stretching burns 3.2 calories.
One minute of sitting while doing nothing else burns 1.1 calories.

ONE YEAR

3.2 calories x 5 days per week = 16 calories

16 calories x 50 weeks per year = 800 calories

800 calories ÷ 3,500 calories per pound = .23 pound

By standing and stretching your hamstrings for one minute per day, instead of sitting, you can burn off almost 1/4 pound per year.

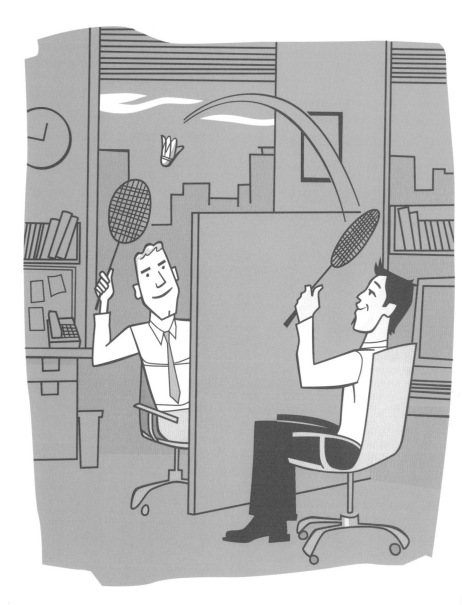

afternoon slump survival

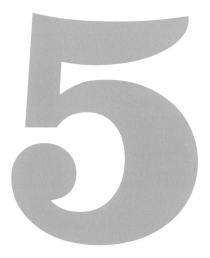

39. computer eye-relief cupping

Staring at your monitor for hours at a time strains and reddens your eyes and blurs your vision. Look away from your computer at least every fifteen minutes and work eye exercises into your daily routine. This exercise soothes and relaxes your eye muscles by warming your eyes and blocking out light.

We never appreciate our vision enough, until we start to lose it. Make time fo this exercise, your eyes will thank you.

> Sit upright with your shoulders relaxed. Rub the palms of your hands together vigorously. While your palms are still warm, lean forward, rest your elbows on your desk, and place your cupped hands lightly over your closed eyes.

> Breathe long, slow, deep breaths as you hold your palms over your eyes for fifteen seconds.

> Uncover your eyes.

> Repeat as necessary to provide relief.

SECRETS OF SUCCESS

Relax and release tension—particularly from the face, neck, and shoulder area—as you breathe deeply. Use the time for a mental break, as well as relief for your eyes. Protect your eyes from computer glare with proper positioning (page 38) and proper lighting.

Eye exercises are not big calorie burners, since the movements are so subtle. You benefit from this exercise by offering some relief to your eyes.

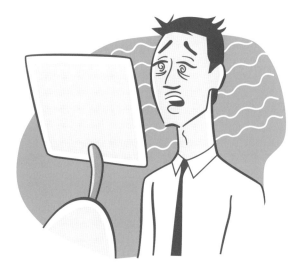

40. look-outside-of-the-box eye-strengthening circles

Strengthen your eye muscles with exercises. Often, we move our head to look in different directions, with very little movement of the eyes. These exercises work the eye muscles to keep them healthy and strong, to prevent eyestrain, and to protect your vision. You may even see something that inspires your next great idea!

> Sit upright with your shoulders relaxed. Keep your head still.

> Breathe normally and maintain good posture as you look up and down three to five times.

> Continue the exercise by looking to the right and left three to five times.

> Circle your eyes in a clockwise direction three to five times, and counterclockwise three to five times.

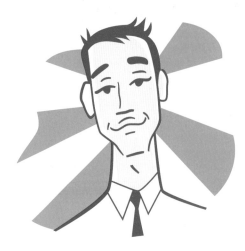

SECRETS OF SUCCESS

If you are self-conscious about rolling your eyes around your head or think that some of your co-workers may get the wrong idea, you can do this exercise with your eyes closed.

Eye exercises are not big calorie burners, since the movements are so subtle. You benefit from these exercises by keeping your eyes strong and healthy.

41. rock-and-roll seated pelvic tilts

There may be constant battling over stations on the office radio, but you can get the rock-and-roll you crave and take care of yourself at the same time. Sitting at your desk can tighten your lower back muscles. Pelvic tilts release lower back tension, condition deep abdominal muscles, and improve pelvic mobility.

Rock and roll to your own inner drummer and keep your back healthy.

> Sit in your chair on your sitz bones with your legs at right angles and space behind your knees.

> Rest your feet on the ground hip-width apart.

> Draw your abdominal muscles inward to support your lower back and keep your pelvis level.

> Lift your breastbone upward as you draw your lower rib cage inward. Align your shoulders above your hips.

> Relax your shoulders. Allow your arms to hang at your sides.

> Inhale as you gently tilt your pelvis forward, arching your lower back slightly.

> Exhale as you pull your navel toward your spine, tilting your pelvis toward the back of your chair.

> Exhale completely, drawing your belly button in toward your spine.

> Repeat for up to one minute.

> Perform exercise as needed during the day to relieve back tension.

One minute of sitting actively burns 2 calories.
One minute of sitting while doing nothing else burns 1.1 calories.

ONE YEAR

2 calories x 5 days per week = 10 calories

10 calories x 50 weeks per year = 500 calories

500 calories ÷ 3,500 calories per pound = .14 pound

By sitting actively for one minute per day, you can burn off more than $1/8$ pound per year.
Clearly, pelvic tilts are not big calorie burners, but this exercise can save your lower back.

42. make-it-to-the-top seated cat stretch

Lower-back pain afflicts more than 85 percent of adults at some point in their life. Keep yourself in the top 15 percent with regular stretching and strengthening exercises. The cat stretch is a classic exercise that keeps your back supple and flexible.

> Sit comfortably in a chair. Place your hands on top of your thighs above your knees.

> Inhale as you look forward and lengthen your spine, stretching from the top of your head to the base of your tailbone.

> Exhale as you look down and round your back, drawing your navel toward your spine, tucking your tailbone under, and spreading your shoulder blades wide.

> Repeat; breathe deeply and flow rhythmically as you round and release your back. Continue for up to one minute.

SECRETS OF SUCCESS
Move through a comfortable range of motion. You should
not feel any pain. Relax and imagine that stress and tension
are flowing out of your body with each exhalation.

One minute of stretching burns 3.2 calories.
One minute of sitting while doing nothing else burns 1.1 calories.

ONE YEAR
3.2 calories x 5 days per week = 16 calories
16 calories x 50 weeks per year = 800 calories
800 calories ÷ 3,500 calories per pound = .23 pound

By adding one minute of desk stretches per day,
you can burn off almost 1/4 pound per year.

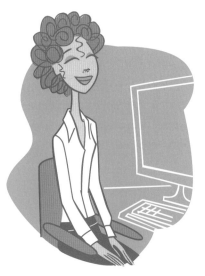

43. "where's my chair?" ab, back, and thigh toner

Read some of your incoming mail as you sit against the wall in your office. Spending a few extra minutes each day in your invisible chair tones up your abs, back, and thighs. Building more muscle mass boosts your metabolism for more calorie burn even while you sleep.

> Stand upright, pressing your back and arms against the wall with your feet hip-width apart, about one foot in front of you. Hold in your abdominal muscles, and relax your shoulders.

> Slide your back down the wall until your thighs are parallel to the floor. Align your knees above your ankles.

> Breathe normally as you hold the seated position. Work for up to one minute.

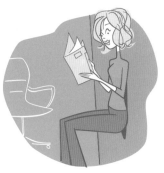

To challenge your abdominal muscles further, slowly lift one foot off the floor and hold for five seconds. Place the foot down. Repeat with the other foot.

SECRETS OF SUCCESS

Start with a five-second hold and gradually increase the length as you grow stronger. If your knees bother you, don't go to a full sitting position. Instead, go approximately halfway down, so your thighs are on a slant rather than parallel to the ground.

One minute of wall-sitting burns 10 calories.
One minute of sitting while doing nothing else burns 1.1 calories.

ONE YEAR

10 calories x 5 days per week = 50 calories

50 calories x 50 weeks per year = 2,500 calories

2,500 calories ÷ 3,500 calories per pound = .71 pound

By adding one minute of wall-sitting per day, instead of sitting at your desk, you can burn off almost ³/₄ pound per year.

44. multitasking seated oblique crunches

Tone your abs while you sit in your chair. Listen for all the compliments on your stunning posture. The most typical way people injure their back is when they bend over and rotate at the waist as they lift or lower something. This exercise strengthens the waist muscles and helps to prevent common back injuries.

» Sit in your chair with good posture (page 36). Keep your hips parallel to your desk. Place your right hand on your right thigh.

» Exhale as you lift your left knee toward your right shoulder and rotate your waist so your right shoulder moves toward your left knee. Avoid rounding your back. Keep your chest lifted and open.

» Inhale as you lower your knee. Continue lifting and lowering left knee for 30 seconds.

» Repeat with your right knee.

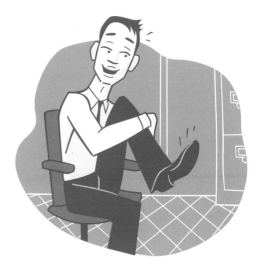

SECRETS OF SUCCESS

Feel the rotation through the muscles of your waist
(imagine squeezing your waist as if you're wringing out a
towel).Do not shift your hips or round your shoulders. Keep
the focus of the exercise on the abdominal muscles.

**One minute of oblique crunches burns 10 calories.
One minute of sitting while doing nothing else burns 1.1 calories.**

ONE YEAR

10 calories x 5 days per week = 50 calories

50 calories x 50 weeks per year = 2,500 calories

2,500 calories ÷ 3,500 calories per pound = .71 pound

By adding one minute of oblique crunches per day, instead of sitting at your desk, you can
burn off almost ³/₄ pound per year and tone up your waist.

45. "is that a cramp in my back?" seated side crunches

Tone your abs while you sit in your chair. Invest only minutes a day at least three times a week on your ab exercises, and you'll see and feel the results after only a few weeks. Once you get stronger, you'll keep it up because you won't want to lose it. You can do it. Focus and be consistent. Make taking care of yourself for a few minutes each day a priority. You are worth it. You deserve to feel your best to get the most out of life.

> Sit in your chair with good posture (page 36). Keep your hips parallel to your desk. Bend your elbows, make soft fists, and hold your fists in front of the center of your chest.

> Exhale as you bend at your waist, lowering your right rib toward your right hipbone and squeezing your abdominal muscles.

> Inhale as you return to the starting position.

> Repeat, alternating sides, and work for up to one minute.

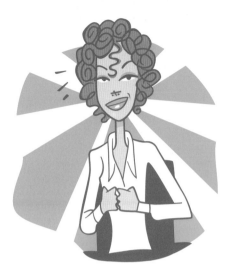

One minute of side crunches burns 10 calories.
One minute of sitting while doing nothing else burns 1.1 calories.

ONE YEAR
10 calories x 5 days per week = 50 calories
50 calories x 50 weeks per year = 2,500 calories
2,500 calories ÷ 3,500 calories per pound = .71 pound

By adding one minute of side crunches per day, instead of sitting at your desk,
you can burn off almost ³/₄ pound per year and tone up your waist.

46. knee-d a break?
seated knee-hug stretch

Take a moment to relieve tension in your lower back. Sitting for long periods of time compresses the spine, particularly the lower back. Enjoy periodic stretches to release muscular tightness. A few minutes of stretching each hour is more effective than thirty minutes all at once (especially when you don't have thirty spare minutes). And you'll feel so much better at the end of the day! Take a few seconds for you.

> Sit comfortably in a chair. Place your hands around the back of your left thigh.

> Exhale as you draw your left knee toward your chest, keeping your right foot on the ground.

> Continue breathing, focusing on the exhalation as you feel a stretch in your buttocks and lower back. Hold for up to thirty seconds.

> Repeat with right leg.

You should not feel any pain. Relax, breathe, and ease slowly into the stretch. Concentrate on the area of the body that you want to stretch. Visualize tension and stress draining out of your body as you exhale. Studies show that keeping a clear mental focus as you exercise leads to better results in a shorter amount of time.

One minute of stretching burns 3.2 calories.
One minute of sitting while doing nothing else burns 1.1 calories.

ONE YEAR

3.2 calories x 5 days per week = 16 calories

16 calories x 50 weeks per year = 800 calories

800 calories ÷ 3,500 calories per pound = .23 pound

By adding one minute of desk stretches per day, you can burn off almost 1/4 pound per year.

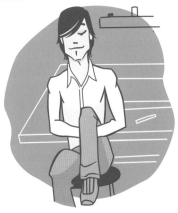

47. this-client-is-a-pain-in-the-buttocks stretch

Deep hip muscles tighten up after sitting for long periods of time—and not just because you had to revise the new client proposal three times. Tight muscles can pinch the sciatic nerve, which can lead to shooting pains down the leg. This stretch can prevent or relieve sciatica by relieving muscle tension. Do it before your pain in the buttocks becomes an even bigger pain in the leg!

➤ Sit comfortably in a chair. Pull your right knee toward your chest and place your right ankle on top of your left thigh. Lean forward from the hips until you feel a stretch deep in your buttocks and hips.

➤ Continue to breathe deeply as you hold the stretch for up to thirty seconds.

➤ Repeat on the other leg.

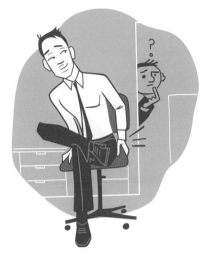

One minute of stretching burns 3.2 calories.
One minute of sitting while doing nothing else burns 1.1 calories.

ONE YEAR
3.2 calories x 5 days per week = 16 calories
16 calories x 50 weeks per year = 800 calories
800 calories ÷ 3,500 calories per pound = .23 pound

By adding one minute of desk stretches per day, you can burn off almost $1/4$ pound
per year.

48. stay-competitive hip and front-of-thigh stretch

The muscles in front of your hips and thighs tighten and shorten after sitting for long periods of time. When these muscles become too tight, they can pull your pelvis forward, causing your lower back to arch and contributing to back strain. This stretch restores length to those muscles—and keeps you focused on doing your best work, instead of on your aching back.

> Sit comfortably on the left edge of your chair with your right foot on the ground. Relax your shoulders.

> Slide the ball of your left foot back on the floor until your left thigh is vertical to the ground with your knee facing down.

> Exhale as you squeeze your buttocks and push the front of your left hip forward. Feel the stretch in the front of your hip and thigh.

> Continue to breathe deeply as you hold the stretch for up to thirty seconds.

> Repeat on the other leg.

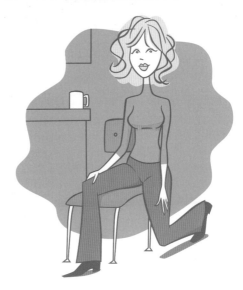

SECRETS OF SUCCESS

Avoid arching your back and keep your chest expanded.
Avoid any feeling of strain in your knees. Focus on feeling
the stretch in the center top of your thighs.

One minute of stretching burns 3.2 calories.
One minute of sitting while doing nothing else burns 1.1 calories.

ONE YEAR

3.2 calories x 5 days per week = 16 calories

16 calories x 50 weeks per year = 800 calories

800 calories ÷ 3,500 calories per pound = .23 pound

By adding a minute per day of desk stretches, you can burn off almost
$^{1}/_{4}$ pound per year.

49. cubicle ab challenge

Perform Olympic-style moves in the comfort of your very own cubicle. This advanced exercise challenges your abs as your strength improves. Be sure to use a sturdy chair that is *not* on rolling wheels.

> Sit in a sturdy and comfortable chair. Place one hand on each side of the seat directly under your shoulders. Stabilize your shoulders by sliding your shoulder blades down.

> Inhale.

> Exhale as you lift your hips up off the seat, tightening your abdominals.

> Inhale as you hold the position.

> Exhale as you lift your knees up toward your chest, feeling a strong contraction in your abdominals.

> Inhale as you lower your knees to the starting position, keeping your hips elevated.

> Repeat as strength permits, working for up to thirty seconds.

One minute of ab challenges burns 10 calories.
One minute of sitting while doing nothing else burns 1.1 calories.

ONE YEAR

10 calories x 5 days per week = 50 calories

50 calories x 50 weeks per year = 2,500 calories

2,500 calories ÷ 3,500 calories per pound = .71 pound

By adding one minute of ab challenges per day,
instead of sitting at your desk, you can burn
off almost 3/4 pound per year and tone
up your waist.

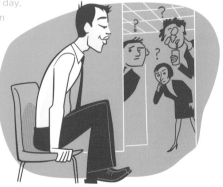

117

50. use-it-or-lose-it inner-thigh toner

Abilities that we don't use, we lose. Scientists now know that many aspects of aging that were thought to be inevitable are simply the result of disuse. Use your abilities to move or lose them. If you do not have a soft five-inch ball to use as a prop, roll up a small towel to squeeze against for resistance. Strong inner thighs help prevent knee pain and add zest to your sex life, which is also important to your health—just be careful with that office romance. And unless you have a glass-top desk, no one knows what you're doing.

> Sit in your chair on your sitz bones with your legs bent at a right angle, space behind your knees, and feet resting on the ground hip-width apart.

> Draw your abdominal muscles inward to support your lower back and keep your pelvis level. Relax your shoulders, allowing your arms to hang at your sides.

> Place a small ball or towel in between your thighs to squeeze against.

> Inhale.

> Exhale as you lift up through the pelvic floor, tighten your abdominals, and squeeze your thighs together, keeping your spinal alignment.

> Inhale; gently relax the pressure without allowing the ball to fall.

> Work for up to one minute.

Keep your head level. Focus the muscle contractions on the pelvic floor, deep abdominals, and inner thighs. Avoid tension in other parts of the body, particularly the neck and shoulders. And keep your eyebrows relaxed. Otherwise, everyone else in the office may raise theirs.

One minute of sitting actively burns 2 calories.
One minute of sitting while doing nothing else burns 1.1 calories.

ONE YEAR

2 calories x 5 days per week = 10 calories
10 calories x 50 weeks per year = 500 calories
500 calories ÷ 3,500 calories per pound = .14 pound

By sitting actively for one minute per day, you can burn off more than 1/8 pound per year. While this exercise is not a big calorie burner, studies show that as people become more fit, their sex life improves. As in all things, use it or lose it!

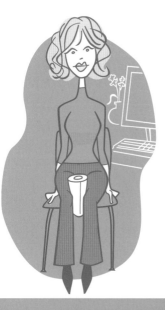

51. toe-the-line seated leg extensions

Toned thighs support your knees, preventing injury and alleviating aches and pains. You can use an ankle weight or tie your exercise band in a circle and place it around your ankles for resistance or, if you prefer to use only the weight of your leg, simply focus on contracting the muscles on the top of the thigh as you perform the exercise. Studies show that people who concentrate on the working muscles tone up more quickly. Train with your brain, not just your body, for optimal results.

> Sit in your chair with good posture (page 36). If you want to use an ankle weight, start with the weight on your right leg. Place a towel underneath the thigh of your weighted leg.

> Draw your abdominal muscles inward to support your lower back and keep your pelvis level. Relax your shoulders, allowing your arms to hang at your sides or holding onto the edge of chair seat.

> Inhale.

> Exhale as you straighten your weighted right leg without locking your knee.

> Inhale as you lower your leg.

> Do eight to twelve repetitions or work for up to one minute.

> Repeat with left leg.

One minute of resisted leg extensions burns 10 calories.
One minute of sitting while doing nothing else burns 1.1 calories.

ONE YEAR

10 calories x 5 days per week = 50 calories

50 calories x 50 weeks per year = 2,500 calories

2,500 calories ÷ 3,500 calories per pound = .71 pound

By adding two minutes of leg extensions per day, instead of simply sitting at your desk,
you can burn off almost 1 1/2 pounds per year and tone up your thighs.

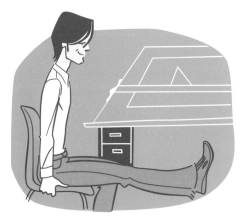

52. board-meeting bun squeezes

Bored with your board meeting? Tone your buttocks during those planning sessions that seem to drag on forever. You can do these silently while seated in your chair.

> Sit in your chair on your sitz bones with your legs bent at a right angle, space behind your knees, and feet resting on the ground hip-width apart.

> Draw your abdominal muscles inward to support your lower back and keep your pelvis level. Relax your shoulders, resting your hands on your thighs with your elbows aligned with your shoulders.

> Inhale.

> Exhale as you squeeze your buttocks muscles, maintaining good posture.

> Inhale and gently relax the muscles.

> Repeat, working for up to one minute.

Keep your head level. Avoid tension in other parts of the
body, particularly the neck and shoulders.

One minute of sitting actively burns 2 calories.
One minute of sitting while doing nothing else burns 1.1 calories.

ONE YEAR
2 calories x 5 days per week = 10 calories
10 calories x 50 weeks per year = 500 calories
500 calories ÷ 3,500 calories per pound = .14 pound

By sitting actively for one minute per day, you can burn off more than ⅛ pound per year.
Any exercises you do to stimulate your buttocks muscles are worth your time. The gluteal
muscles are the largest muscle group in the body. More lean body mass equals a higher
metabolic rate, which means more calorie-burning even when you sleep.

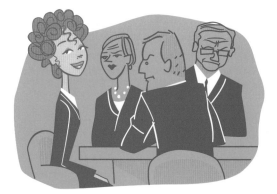

53. listen-to-your-voice-mail standing side leg lifts

Take a break from sitting. Stand and listen to your voice-mail messages while you tone and strengthen your outer thighs. You can use an ankle weight, exercise band, or the weight of your leg for resistance. Strong thigh muscles stabilize the knee joint and help prevent knee pain.

» Stand upright, hold in your abdominal muscles, and relax your shoulders.

» Place your left hand on a chair, desk, filing cabinet, or wall for support.

» Stand on your left leg. If using an ankle weight, put it on the right leg.

» Exhale as you lift your right leg to the side as high as possible without losing alignment. Keep your foot and kneecap facing forward. Avoid tilting your hips forward or hiking up your right hip. Lift up the pelvic floor muscles and tighten your deep abdominals to help stabilize the pelvis.

» Inhale as you return to the starting position.

» Continue for thirty seconds.

» Switch legs and repeat.

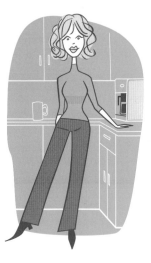

Stabilize your posture by contracting your deep abdominal muscles. Breathe smoothly and avoid holding tension in other parts of the body.

One minute of resisted side leg lifts burns 10 calories.
One minute of standing burns 2 calories.

ONE YEAR

10 calories x 5 days per week = 50 calories

50 calories x 50 weeks per year = 2,500 calories

2,500 calories ÷ 3,500 calories per pound = .71 pound

By adding one minute of side leg lifts per day, instead of simply sitting in your cubicle, you can burn off almost ³/₄ pound per year and tone up your thighs.

54. circulation-boosting standing leg curls

Sitting for hours in a chair diminishes the blood flow to your lower body. Some people even experience foot pain, swelling, or leg cramps. Boost your circulation and tone the muscles in the backs of your thighs with this exercise. Use an ankle weight or tie your exercise band in a circle and place it around your ankle for more resistance and better results.

> Stand facing a wall or piece of furniture, hold in your abdominals, and relax your shoulders.

> Place your hands on the wall or a piece of furniture for support.

> Stand on your right leg. If using an ankle weight or exercise band, put it around the left leg.

> Keep your knees next to each other and your thighs in a vertical line. Exhale as you bend your left knee and pull your heel toward your buttocks without losing your alignment. Avoid arching your lower back. Lift up the pelvic floor muscles and tighten your deep abdominals to stabilize the pelvis.

> Inhale as you return to the starting position.

> Continue for thirty seconds.

> Switch legs and repeat.

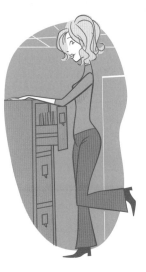

SECRETS OF SUCCESS

Stabilize your posture by using the deep abdominal and pelvic-floor muscles. Relax your jaw, neck, and shoulders. Tone up your abs by keeping your torso as still as possible, moving only your leg.

One minute of resisted leg curls burns 10 calories.
One minute of standing burns 2 calories.

. . . .

ONE YEAR

10 calories x 5 days per week = 50 calories

50 calories x 50 weeks per year = 2,500 calories

2,500 calories ÷ 3,500 calories per pound = .71 pound

By adding one minute of inner-thigh crossovers per day, instead of simply standing in your cubicle, you can burn off almost ³/₄ pound per year and tone up your thighs.

55. hit-your-target chair triceps dips

Unless you're moving office furniture, you're not likely to use your triceps, the muscles in the backs of your upper arms. Tone up your arms and the muscles that stabilize your shoulder joints with chair dips. Strong shoulder joints help prevent shoulder injuries, especially when you lift and reach for items. Technology eliminates most of the need to do any physical labor, including pushing things. That's why you need to strategize to add extra movement and exercises into your day. Create daily goals such as promising yourself that you will do at least five exercises per day. Then, hit your target.

> Sit on the edge of a sturdy chair that can support your weight and does not have wheels or a slippery seat that you cannot grip securely. Place your feet on the floor several inches in front of your knees. Place your hands on the edge of the seat directly under your shoulders.

> Slide your shoulder blades down to stabilize your shoulders. Slide your hips off the front of the chair.

> Inhale.

> Exhale as you bend your elbows until they are almost up to shoulder height, lowering your hips toward the floor.

> Inhale and hold the position.

> Exhale as you push up to the starting position.

> Do eight to twelve repetitions or work for up to one minute.

One minute of triceps dips burns 10 calories.
One minute of sitting while doing nothing else burns 1.1 calories.

ONE YEAR

10 calories x 5 days per week = 50 calories
50 calories x 50 weeks per year = 2,500 calories
2,500 calories ÷ 3,500 calories per pound = .71 pound

By adding one minute of triceps dips per day, you can burn off almost $3/4$ pound per year
and tone up your upper arms.

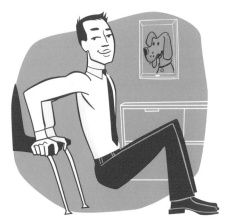

56. action-item tele-stretch

Put self-care at the top of your action-item list and everything else will get done faster. Talking for long hours on the phone can strain the neck and shoulders and lead to a tilting posture if you do not have a headset. Avoid muscle tension and take advantage of using a handheld receiver by changing sides and enjoying a neck stretch. Just be sure to remember to alternate sides so you don't create a posture with a tilting head.

> Sit with good posture with your shoulders relaxed and your arms at your sides (page 36).

> Keep your hips and feet facing your desk.

> Lower your right ear toward your shoulder. Place the phone under your right ear and place your right hand at your side. Keep your face forward and chin level. Avoid arching the back of your neck.

> Breathe deeply as you hold the stretch for up to thirty seconds.

> Repeat on the other side.

SECRETS OF SUCCESS
Avoid forcing a stretch. Instead, ease gently into an
increased range of motion, stretching only to a moderate
point of tension.

One minute of stretching burns 3.2 calories.
One minute of sitting while doing nothing else burns 1.1 calories.

ONE YEAR

3.2 calories x 5 days per week = 16 calories

16 calories x 50 weeks per year = 800 calories

800 calories ÷ 3,500 calories per pound = .23 pound

By adding one minute of desk stretches per day, you can burn off almost ¼ pound per
year. Keep in mind that the value of these smaller exercises is in creating good posture,
balancing muscle development, and feeling better. You are only as strong as your weakest
link. If your abs are very strong and your neck muscles are weak, your posture lacks
balance. Seek harmony and balance in all things for the best results.

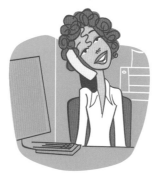

57. productivity-increasing tele-stroll

Take advantage of phone meetings to stroll back and forth while wearing your wireless headset. Your telephone colleagues will be none the wiser. The circulatory boost may even inspire clearer thinking, new ideas, and better productivity. If you don't have a cordless headset, consider getting one. It will help you maintain good posture.

> Stand with good posture (page 42).

> Pull in your abdominal muscles slightly to support your lower back. Relax your shoulders.

> Swing your arms naturally at your sides with your palms facing in.

> Walk at a gentle pace so that you can easily carry on a telephone conversation.

> Maintain a pace of less than a twenty-minute mile.

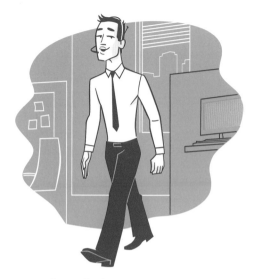

When you perform turns during your pacing, maintain good posture. If it is not possible to pace, then stand during conversations, rather than sit.

One minute of strolling burns 3.8 calories.
One minute of standing burns 2 calories.

ONE YEAR

3.8 calories x 5 days per week = 19 calories

19 calories x 50 weeks per year = 950 calories

950 calories ÷ 3,500 calories per pound = .27 pound

By adding four minutes of strolling per day, you can burn off up to 1 pound per year. And never underestimate how much you can increase your productivity when you have more energy and feel refreshed and clear-minded. Working while healthy is good for you *and* good for business.

58. "all in favor say aye" reverse curls

Raise your hand in favor of strong muscles and a healthy body. Reverse curls tone the front of your upper arms and condition your wrists and forearms. Strong forearms prevent wrist strain from long stints at the keyboard. Use a weighted water bottle for resistance, or simply concentrate and tighten the targeted muscles. Do this exercise standing or sitting.

- Stand holding a weighted water bottle in your left hand, with your arms hanging at your sides, palms facing back, and shoulders relaxed. Your feet should be hip-width apart.

- Exhale as you bend your left elbow and lift up the weight to shoulder height with your palm facing out. Keep your wrist flat. Squeeze your biceps muscle when the weight is at its highest point.

- Inhale as you lower the weight back to the starting position.

- Continue for eight to twelve repetitions or for thirty seconds.

- Switch sides and repeat.

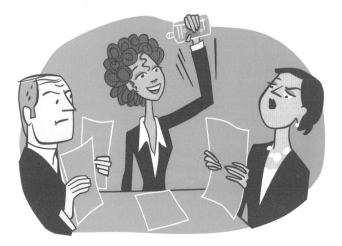

Use your core muscles and tighten your abdominals to keep
your posture strong. Avoid arching your back or rocking
back and forth.

One minute of reverse curls burns 10 calories.
One minute of standing burns 2 calories.

ONE YEAR
10 calories x 5 days per week = 50 calories
50 calories x 50 weeks per year = 2,500 calories
2,500 calories ÷ 3,500 calories per pound = .71 pound

By adding one minute of standing reverse curls per day, instead of simply standing, you
can burn off almost ³/₄ pound per year and tone up your arms.

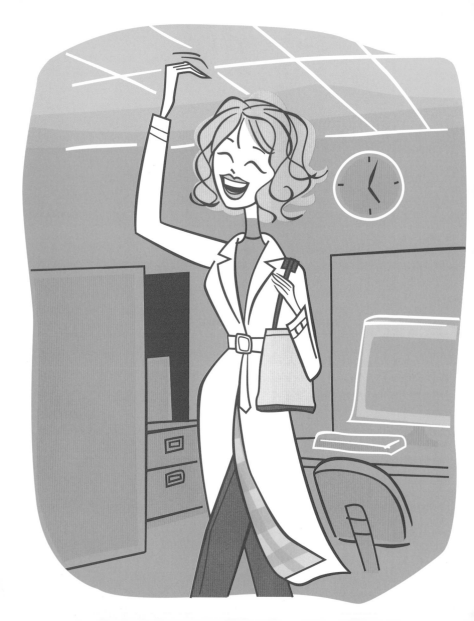

evening stress busters

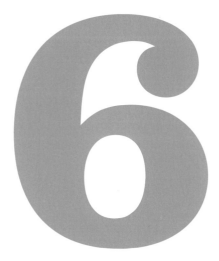

59. day-is-done overhead presses

Sometimes you just want to shout *hooray* at the end of the workday. Celebrate the moment with a set of overhead presses to tone and strengthen your shoulders and condition the muscles that support your shoulder joints and help you have good posture. Use weighted water bottles for resistance. Do this exercise seated or standing.

> Sit comfortably in your chair with your shoulders relaxed, your arms at your sides, holding a weighted water bottle in each hand. Tighten your abdominal muscles to support your back. Maintain good posture (page 36).

> Lift your hands to shoulder height, elbows bent, palms facing forward.

> Exhale as you push both arms up overhead, palms facing forward. Keep your shoulders relaxed, torso stable, and wrists flat. Avoid hunching your shoulders or arching your lower back.

> Inhale as you lower your arms to the starting position.

> Do eight to twelve repetitions or work for thirty seconds.

> Switch arms and repeat.

One minute of overhead presses burns 10 calories.
One minute of sitting while doing nothing else burns 1.1 calories.

ONE YEAR

10 calories x 5 days per week = 50 calories
50 calories x 50 weeks per year = 2,500 calories
2,500 calories ÷ 3,500 calories per pound = .71 pound

By adding one minute of overhead presses
per day, you can burn off almost ³/₄ pound
per year and tone up your shoulders.

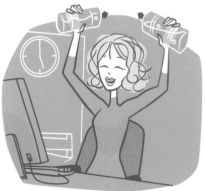

60. clear-the-air rear-shoulder squeeze

Clear the air around your desk and cubicle as you prepare to head home. Use an exercise band or simply tighten the targeted muscles for resistance to tone up the back of your shoulders. Avoid a slouched posture by balancing the strength of the front and back of your shoulders. Do this exercise seated or standing.

- Sit comfortably in your chair, shoulders relaxed, arms at sides, holding a band in front of your body or a weighted water bottle in your right hand. Tighten your abdominals to support your back. Maintain good posture (page 36).

- Lift your right arm up to shoulder height, keeping your wrist flat and your shoulders relaxed.

- Exhale as you sweep your right arm back and straight out to the side at shoulder height. Keep your shoulders relaxed, torso stable, and wrist flat.

- Inhale as you return your arm to the starting position.

- Do eight to twelve repetitions or work for thirty seconds.

- Switch arms and repeat.

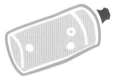

**One minute of standing rear shoulder squeezes burns 10 calories.
One minute of sitting while doing nothing else burns 1.1 calories.**

ONE YEAR

10 calories x 5 days per week = 50 calories

50 calories x 50 weeks per year = 2,500 calories

2,500 calories ÷ 3,500 calories per pound = .71 pound

By adding one minute of rear shoulder squeezes per day, instead of simply sitting at your desk, you can burn off almost ³/₄ pound per year and tone up your shoulders.

61. "ask for a raise!" forward raises

Let others think you're staying late again, angling for a big promotion. Toning up your shoulders helps prevent injuries and creates a strong shoulder line. Use an exercise band or weighted water bottle for resistance. Do this exercise seated or standing. Drink up the water in your bottle in between exercises and fit in an extra stroll to the drinking fountain to fill it up again before your next round of exercise. Keep thinking of ways to move more each day.

> Sit comfortably in your chair with your shoulders relaxed and your arms at your sides, holding the exercise band in front of your body with one end of the band in each hand. Place your left hand at your waist and your right hand at your side with your right wrist flat and palm facing back. Tighten your abdominals to support your back. Maintain good posture (page 36).

> Exhale as you lift your right arm forward up to shoulder height, keeping your shoulders relaxed, torso stable, and wrist flat. Avoid hunching your shoulders or rotating your torso.

> Inhale as you lower your arm to the starting position.

> Do eight to twelve repetitions or work for thirty seconds.

> Switch arms and repeat.

Do not do this exercise if you experience any back, shoulder, or wrist pain. Strengthen your forearms first with wrist exercises (page 74) and reverse curls (page 16). Feel the exercise in your shoulders.

One minute of sitting forward raises burns 10 calories.
One minute of sitting while doing nothing else burns 1.1 calories.

ONE YEAR

10 calories x 5 days per week = 50 calories
50 calories x 50 weeks per year = 2,500 calories
2,500 calories ÷ 3,500 calories per pound = .71 pound

By adding one minute of forward raises per day, you can burn off almost ³/₄ pound per year and tone up your shoulders.

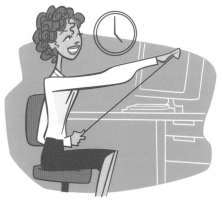

62. take-off-your-game-face self-massage

Tension often gets stored in facial muscles, which can contribute to a tired and unhappy expression. Refresh and relax yourself, while restoring a more youthful appearance with simple self-massage techniques. The increased circulation also improves your skin's tone and complexion.

> Sit upright with your shoulders relaxed, maintaining good posture (page 36). Rub the palms of your hands together vigorously. While your palms are still warm, place your hands on the surface of your face to warm the skin.

> Cup your hands, holding fingers wide apart.

> Place the pads of your fingertips all around your hairline, gently pressing and releasing. Breathe deeply, releasing tension with each exhalation.

> Continue pressing the pads of your fingertips on your eyebrows and around the eye bones.

> Gently trace under your cheekbones with your thumbs, pressing and releasing.

> Using the pads of your index and middle fingers, trace, press, and release around your nose.

> With your thumbs and index fingers, squeeze your chin and trace the jawline. Gently massage under your ears at the jaw joints.

> Finish by taking a big yawn, opening your eyes wide, and stretching your jaw. If you're not embarrassed, stick your tongue out as far as it will go to stretch and relax the back of your throat. Just make sure you're not looking at a colleague.

One minute of sitting actively burns 2 calories.
One minute of sitting while doing nothing else burns 1.1 calories.

ONE YEAR

2 calories x 5 days per week = 10 calories

10 calories x 50 weeks per year = 500 calories

500 calories ÷ 3,500 calories per pound = .14 pound

By sitting actively for one minute per day, you can burn off a little more than $1/_8$ pound per year.

63. "file under f for fabulous" scalp self-massage

Office stress can even get stored in your scalp. And tight muscles impair good circulation, which is necessary for healthy hair. To feel great and ensure good circulation for a healthy head of hair, enjoy this scalp self-massage.

> Sit upright with your shoulders relaxed, maintaining good posture (page 36). Cup your hands, holding your fingers wide apart.

> Place the pads of your fingertips all around your scalp, gently pressing and releasing. Breathe deeply, releasing tension with each exhalation.

> Place your hands on either side of your scalp and move the scalp back and forth, as if it were a hairpiece. Move the skin and muscles, and keep your fingers in the same spots. Reposition your hands all around the scalp and hairline and repeat.

> Finish with a shampooing movement. Vigorously move the pads of your fingertips back and forth on various spots on your head, creating friction and heat. Imagine washing that office stress right out of your hair.

> Breathe deeply and enjoy the sense of relief and invigoration when you are finished.

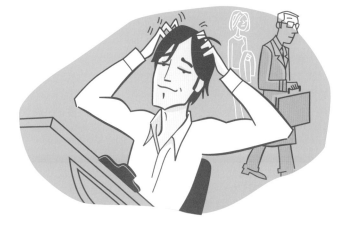

One minute of sitting actively burns 2 calories.
One minute of sitting while doing nothing else burns 1.1 calories.

ONE YEAR

2 calories x 5 days per week = 10 calories

10 calories x 50 weeks per year = 500 calories

500 calories ÷ 3,500 calories per pound = .14 pound

By sitting actively for one minute per day, you can burn off more than ¹/₈ pound per year.

64. tension-busting shoulder self-massage

If you have time for only one exercise to release stress and tension, this is it. You can do this effective self-massage anytime during the day when you feel tight in the shoulders or at night, before you go to sleep, to help you unwind.

> Sit upright with your shoulders relaxed, maintaining good posture (page 36). Cup your hands, holding your fingers close together.

> Reach across your body with your right hand and place the pads of your right fingertips on the back of your shoulder line with your thumb on the front and your palm touching the shoulder. Pinch the thumb and fingertips toward each other, squeezing the muscle on top of your shoulder. Breathe deeply and hold for ten to fifteen seconds. If your shoulders are very tight, you may feel tension moving up into your temple.

> Repeat two or three times. Feel the tension decrease with each repetition.

> Squeeze and release the muscle on top of your shoulder several times, moving your hand along the shoulder and grabbing as much flesh as you can.

- Reach back with your right hand down your back and spread your fingertips wide. Rake upward, feeling the muscles underneath. Continue raking, reaching in as many directions as possible.

- Relax and repeat on the other side.

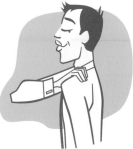

SECRETS OF SUCCESS

This area can be extremely tight and even painful for some people. Work gently and breathe deeply. You will be amazed at how much tension you can release.

One minute of sitting actively burns 2 calories.
One minute of sitting while doing nothing else burns 1.1 calories.

ONE YEAR

2 calories x 5 days per week = 10 calories
10 calories x 50 weeks per year = 500 calories
500 calories ÷ 3,500 calories per pound = .14 pound

By sitting actively for one minute per day, you can burn off more than 1/8 pound per year. By reducing tension in your body, you can also lower feelings of mental tension and stress. Studies show that stress is a factor in 80 percent of the most common diseases and contributes to poorer health. Long, slow, deep breaths reduce your heart rate and blood pressure and restore feelings of balance and well-being. Take time to breathe and relax, so you can live longer and enjoy life more.

65. keyboard-relief arm and hand self-massage

At the end of a long day typing at your computer, your arms and hands deserve welcome relief. Help prevent repetitive-motion injuries with this easy self-massage. It's the perfect way to end your workday and leave your workstation—and work worries—behind.

> Sit upright with your shoulders relaxed, maintaining good posture (page 36). Use your right hand to squeeze and release your left arm from the shoulder all the way down to the hand. Use gentle pressure as you place the full palm against the arm repeatedly. Repeat three times.

> Use your right thumb to scrub all around the left wrist as if you are washing it.

> Place the thumb in between the knuckles on top of your hand, and the pads of your index and middle fingers on the palm directly underneath the thumb. With gentle pressure, trace lines from the knuckles to the wrist joint. Repeat between all of the knuckles.

> With your right thumb and index finger, gently squeeze in between the thumb and index finger.

> Turn your left palm up. Using the pad of your thumb, scrub the hand from the base of each finger down to the wrist and all around the palm.

- With your right hand, take each finger and the thumb of your left hand and squeeze it as if you are washing it from the base of the finger to the tip.

- Repeat on the other side.

One minute of sitting actively burns 2 calories.
One minute of sitting while doing nothing else burns 1.1 calories.

ONE YEAR

2 calories x 5 days per week = 10 calories

10 calories x 50 weeks per year = 500 calories

500 calories ÷ 3,500 calories per pound = .14 pound

By sitting actively for one minute per day, you can burn off more than 1/8 pound per year. Relaxing may not be a calorie-burning activity, but it can contribute to successful weight management. High levels of stress contribute to storing fat in the abdominal area. Unmanaged stress also triggers emotional eating and reaching for high-fat, high-sugar comfort foods. Make time to wind down because you deserve to feel good.

66. glide-into-the-weekend chin glides

Practice chin glides as you wait in traffic and keep fellow commuters guessing. You may resemble a clucking chicken while you do this exercise, but you will benefit from strengthening your neck muscles. Your head weighs anywhere from eight to twelve pounds. Holding your head erect with your ears aligned above your shoulders is key to good posture and reduces neck and shoulder tension. Sitting for long hours at a time contributes to tight, weak neck muscles. Add these strengthening exercises, and you will feel a world of difference.

》 Sit upright with your shoulders relaxed and your arms at your sides.

》 Exhale as you gently flatten the curve in the back of your neck by drawing your chin back and in, as if you're making a double chin. Keep your chin level. Do not drop your head forward.

》 Inhale as you return to the starting position.

》 Imagine that you are growing taller by creating length in the back of your neck.

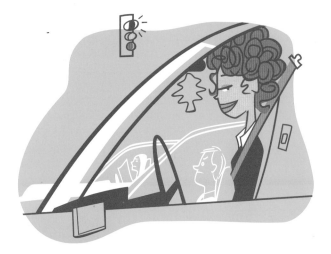

One minute of sitting actively burns 2 calories.
One minute of sitting while doing nothing else burns 1.1 calories.

ONE YEAR

2 calories x 5 days per week = 10 calories

10 calories x 50 weeks per year = 500 calories

500 calories ÷ 3,500 calories per pound = .14 pound

By sitting actively for one minute per day, you can burn off a little more than
1/8 pound per year.

67. "the stock price is climbing!" neck press

Make your fellow commuters crazy with curiosity while you enjoy stretching. Exaggerate your facial expressions as you press your hands to your head. Everyone will wonder what surprising news you have just heard.

> Sit upright with your shoulders relaxed.

> Place the palms of both hands behind your head.

> Exhale as you push the back of your head into your hands with backward resistance as you press your hands forward for an isometric contraction. Hold for six to eight seconds.

> Repeat five to six times.

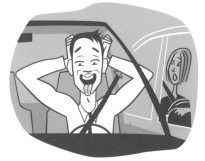

One minute of sitting actively burns 2 calories.
One minute of sitting while doing nothing else burns 1.1 calories.

ONE YEAR

2 calories x 5 days per week = 10 calories

10 calories x 50 weeks per year = 500 calories

500 calories ÷ 3,500 calories per pound = .14 pound

By sitting actively for one minute per day, you can burn off a little more than $1/8$ pound per year.

68. traveling-gym external-rotators toner

You have so much to do now in your traveling gym on your way home that you'll be hoping for gridlock. Strengthen your shoulder muscles and keep your shoulder joints healthy with this external-rotators toner. If you're not embarrassed, you can hold an exercise band in your hands in front of your body.

» Sit upright with your shoulders relaxed and your upper arms against your torso.

» Bend your elbows at a 90-degree angle, with your hands forward and palms facing up.

» Exhale as you open your arms out to the sides as you keep your elbows against your waist.

» Keep your shoulders relaxed as you feel the muscles working under your armpits, close to your ribs.

» Inhale as you return your arms to the starting position.

One minute of sitting actively burns 2 calories.
One minute of sitting while doing nothing else burns 1.1 calories.

ONE YEAR

2 calories x 5 days per week = 10 calories

10 calories x 50 weeks per year = 500 calories

500 calories ÷ 3,500 calories per pound = .14 pound

By sitting actively for one minute per day, you can burn off a little more than
1/8 pound per year.

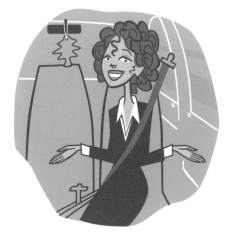

69. "where's the party?" ankle taps

Get in the party mood as you head home. When you're waiting in traffic, tap away to your favorite tunes and feel the rhythm. Ankle taps tone your shins and condition your ankles. This exercise helps you to walk comfortably. Walking is one of the best exercises for improving your health, and one you can enjoy your entire life.

> Sit upright with your shoulders relaxed and your arms at your sides.

> If you're in the car, be sure to keep one foot on the brake.

> With your free foot, lift and lower the ball of the foot as you keep your heel on the ground.

> After ten taps, switch to taps that alternate from one side of your foot to the other as you lift the ball of your foot and rotate your ankle.

> Lift the ball of your foot as high as you can by flexing your shin.

> Repeat with your other foot.

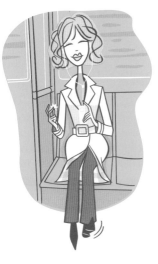

One minute of sitting actively burns 2 calories.
One minute of sitting while doing nothing else burns 1.1 calories.

ONE YEAR

2 calories x 5 days per week = 10 calories

10 calories x 50 weeks per year = 500 calories

500 calories ÷ 3,500 calories per pound = .14 pound

By sitting actively for one minute per day, you can burn off a little more than
$^1/_8$ pound per year.

acknowledgments

Thanks very much to my many corporate students for helping me to be a better workplace wellness teacher and for desk-testing the exercises and providing great feedback. A big thank you to Jodi Davis and Lisa Campbell at Chronicle Books for their support. Thanks also to Chuck Gonzales, the illustrator, for breathing life and energy into our office "models" and to the Chronicle art team for doing such a beautiful job. A very special thanks and big hugs to Georgia Archer and Anthony Dominici for their love, support, honest opinions, and encouragement. —SA

. . . .

Illustrator Biography

Chuck Gonzales is a New York City–based artist whose clients include the *Wall Street Journal, New York Times, Newsweek,* and numerous other publications. His work has been featured on MTV and he has also designed characters and backgrounds for a Nickelodeon cartoon.